MW01041147

USMLE®

STEP 1

Lecture Notes

2017

Behavioral Science and Social Sciences

Published by Kaplan Medical, a division of Kaplan, Inc.
750 Third Avenue
New York, NY 10017
10 9 8 7 6 5 4 3 2 1

Course ISBN: 978-1-5062-0871-8

Retail ISBN: 978-1-5062-0834-3

Editors

Epidemiology, Statistics, Behavioral Science

Charles Faselis, M.D.
Chairman of Medicine
VA Medical Center
Washington, DC

Alina Gonzalez-Mayo, M.D.
Psychiatrist
Department of Veterans Administration
Bay Pines, FL

Mark Tyler-Lloyd, M.D., M.P.H.
Executive Director of Academics
Kaplan Medical
New York, NY

Basic Science of Patient Safety

Ted A. James, M.D., M.S., F.A.C.S.
Chief, Breast Surgical Oncology
Vice Chair, Academic Affairs
Department of Surgery
Beth Israel Deaconess Medical Center
Harvard Medical School
Boston, MA

We want to hear what you think. What do you like or not like about the Notes?
Please email us at **medfeedback@kaplan.com**.

Contents

SECTION I

Epidemiology and Biostatistics

Epidemiology 1

Learning Objectives

- ❏ Answer questions about epidemiologic measures
- ❏ Use knowledge of screening tests
- ❏ Explain information related to study designs

EPIDEMIOLOGIC MEASURES

Epidemiology is the study of the distribution and determinants of health-related states within a population. It refers to the patterns of disease and the factors that influence those patterns.

- **Endemic**: the usual, expected rate of disease over time; the disease is maintained without much variation within a region
- **Epidemic**: occurrence of disease in excess of the expected rate; usually presents in a larger geographic span than endemics (*epidemiology* is the study of epidemics)
- **Pandemic**: worldwide epidemic
- **Epidemic curve**: visual description (commonly histogram) of an epidemic curve is disease cases plotted against time; classic signature of an epidemic is a "spike" in time

The tools of epidemiology are numbers; the numbers in epidemiology are ratios converted into rates. The denominator is key: who is "at risk" for a particular event or disease state.

To determine the rate, compare the number of actual cases with the number of potential cases:

$$\frac{\text{Actual cases}}{\text{Potential cases}} = \frac{\text{Numerator}}{\text{Denominator}} = \text{RATE}$$

Rates are generally, though not always, per 100,000 persons by the Centers for Disease Control (CDC), but can be per any multiplier. (Vital statistics are usually per 1,000 persons.)

A disease may occur in a country at a regular annual rate, which makes it **endemic**. If there is a sudden rise in the number of cases in a specific month, we say that there is an **epidemic**. As the disease continues to rise and spread to other countries, it becomes a **pandemic**. Thus the terminology is related to both the number of cases and its geographical distribution.

The graph below represents the incidence of 2 diseases (cases in 100,000). Disease 1 is endemic as the rate of disease is consistent month to month with minor variation in the number of cases. Disease 2 experiences an epidemic in March and April in which the number of cases is in excess of what is expected.

January	February	March	April	May	June	July	August
3	4	3	4	4	4	3	3
5	5	8	8	5	5	5	5

Although the data is in 100,000 cases, the variation in disease 1 is still consistent when compared to disease 2.

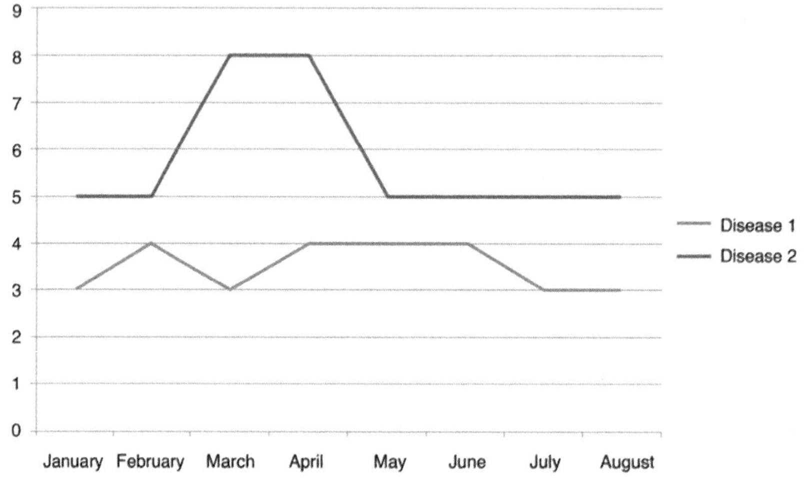

Figure 1.1 Epidemic vs. Endemic Cases

Consider the following scenario. A Japanese farmer begins to sell meat that is infected with salmonella. Within 2 days, hundreds of villagers begin to experience crampy abdominal pain. This is an example of an epidemic. The sudden rise of salmonella gastroenteritis in this village is much higher than the average incidence for the given time period.

Now what if the farmer ships 1,000 pounds of infected beef to other regions of Japan before he realizes what happened. What can one anticipate would happen? The answer is there would be no change to the endemic rate of gastroenteritis. The farmer is only shipping out 1,000 pounds of beef to a few cities nationwide. Unlike the earlier scenario which addressed the population of a village, this would be the entire nation. Assuming that every person who consumes the beef gets gastroenteritis, that number would not significantly increase the national average of cases and would therefore not significantly change the incidence of the disease nationwide.

Incidence and Prevalence

Incidence rate (IR) is the rate at which **new events** occur in a population.

- The numerator is the number of **new** events that occur in a defined period.
- The denominator is the population at risk of experiencing this new event during the same period.

$$\text{Incidence rate} = \frac{\text{Number of new events in a specified period}}{\text{Number of persons "exposed to risk" of becoming new cases during this period}} \times 10^n$$

The IR includes only **new cases** of the disease that occurred during the specified period, not cases that were diagnosed earlier. This is especially important when working with infectious diseases such as TB and malaria.

If, over the course of a year, 5 men are diagnosed with prostate cancer, out of a total male study population of 200 (with no prostate cancer at the beginning of the study period), the IR of prostate cancer in this population would be 0.025 (or 2,500 per 100,000 men-years of study).

Attack rate is the cumulative incidence of infection in a group of people observed over a period of time during an epidemic, usually in relation to food-borne illness. It is measured from the beginning of an outbreak to the end of the outbreak.

$$\text{Attack rate} = \frac{\text{Number of exposed people infected with the disease}}{\text{Total number of exposed people}}$$

Attack rate is also called *attack ratio*; consider an outbreak of Norwalk virus in which 18 people in separate households become ill. If the population of the community is 1,000, the overall attack rate is $\frac{18}{1,000} \times 100\% = 1.8\%$.

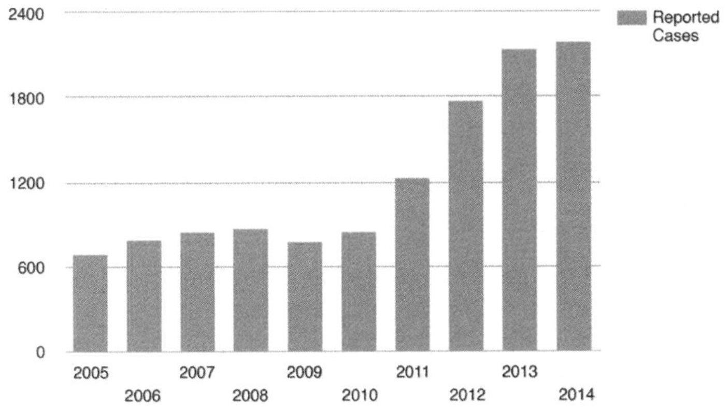

Figure 1.2 Reported Cases of Hepatitis C in the United States

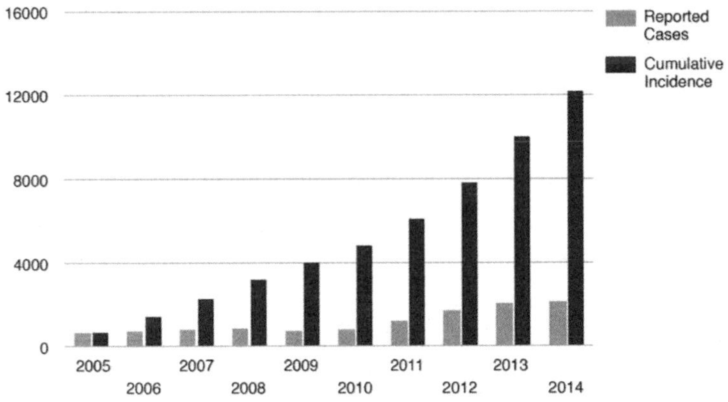

Figure 1.3 Cumulative Incidence 2005–2015

Prevalence is all persons who experience an event in a population. The numerator is all individuals who have an attribute or disease at a particular point in time (or period of time). The denominator is the population at risk of having the attribute or disease at that point in time or midway through the period.

$$\text{Prevalence} = \frac{\text{All cases of a disease at a given point / period}}{\text{Total population “at risk” for being cases at a given point / period}} \times 10^n$$

Prevalence, in other words, is the proportion of people in a population who have a particular disease at a specified point in time (or over a specified period of time). The numerator includes both new cases and old cases (people who remained ill during the specified point or period in time). A case is counted in prevalence until death or recovery occurs. **This makes prevalence different from incidence, which includes only new cases in the numerator.**

Prevalence is most useful for measuring the burden of chronic disease in a population, such as TB, malaria and HIV. For example, the CDC estimated the prevalence of obesity among American adults in 2001 at approximately 20%. Since the number (20%) includes all cases of obesity in the United States, we are talking about *prevalence*.

Note

Prevalence is a measurement of *all* individuals (new and old) affected by the disease at a particular time, whereas **incidence** is a measurement of the number of *new* individuals who contract a disease during a particular period of time.

Point prevalence is useful for comparing disease at different points in time in order to determine whether an outbreak is occurring. We know that the amount of disease present in a population changes over time, but we may need to know how much of a particular disease is present in a population at a single point in time (“snapshot view”).

Perhaps we want to know the prevalence of TB in Community A today. To do that, we need to calculate the point prevalence on a given date. The numerator would include all known TB patients who live in Community A that day. The denominator would be the population of Community A that day.

Period prevalence, on the other hand, is prevalence during a specified period or span of time. The focus is on *chronic* conditions.

In the **“prevalence pot,”** incident (or new) cases are monitored over time. New cases join pre-existing cases to make up total prevalence.

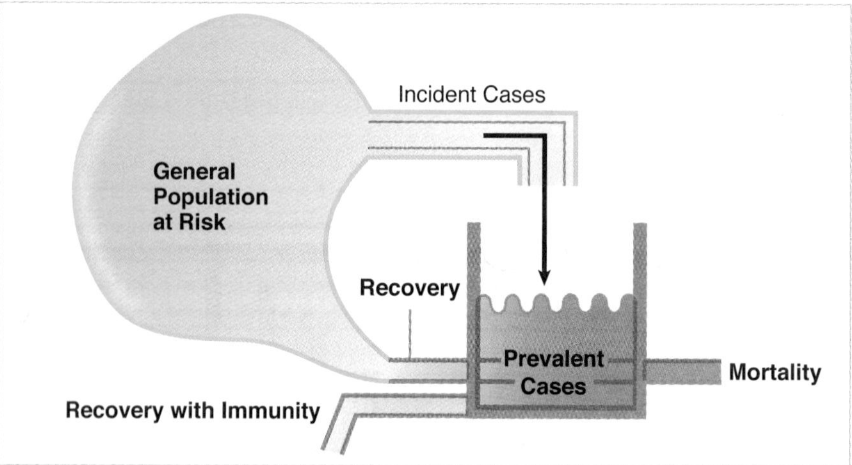

Figure 1-4. Prevalence Pot

Prevalent cases leave the prevalence pot in one of 2 ways: recovery or death.

Table 1-1. Incidence and Prevalence

What happens if:	Incidence	Prevalence
New effective treatment is initiated	no change	decrease
New effective vaccine gains widespread use	decrease	decrease
Number of persons dying from the condition increases	no change	decrease
Additional Federal research dollars are targeted to a specific condition	no change	no change
Behavioral risk factors are reduced in the population at large	decrease	decrease
Contacts between infected persons and noninfected persons are reduced		
For airborne infectious disease?	decrease	decrease
For noninfectious disease?	no change	no change
Recovery from the disease is more rapid than it was 1 year ago	no change	decrease
Long-term survival rates for the disease are increasing	no change	increase

Note

Morbidity rate is the rate of disease in a population at risk (for both incident and prevalent cases), while **mortality rate** is the rate of death in a population at risk (incident cases only).

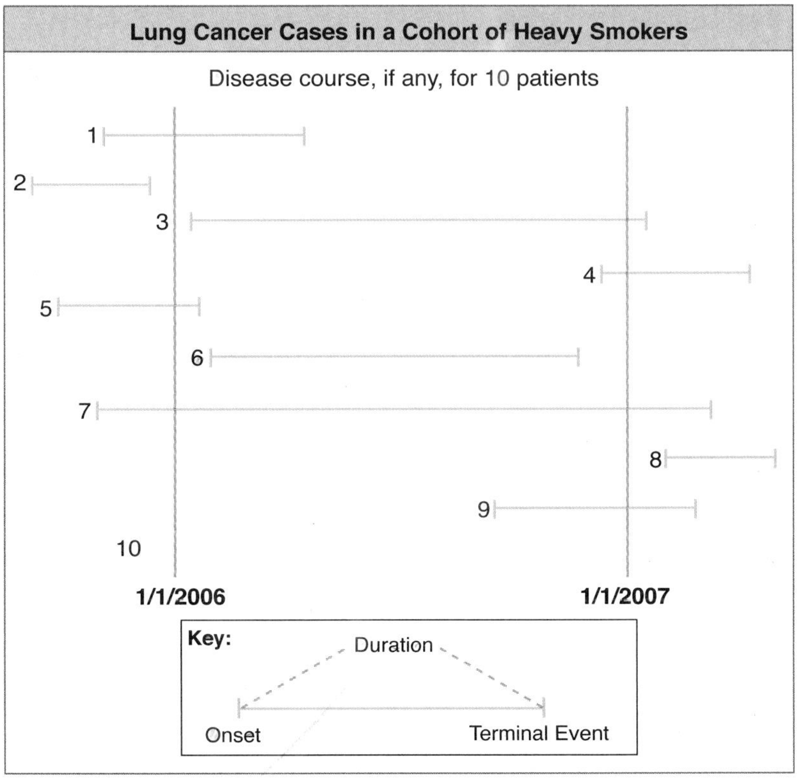

Figure 1-5. Calculating Incidence and Prevalence

Based on the graph above, calculate the following:

- **Prevalence of lung cancer from 1/1/2016–1/1/2017**
  - Number of patients who "had" lung cancer in this time period from the graph: (7)
  - Number of patients at risk in this time period: (9) [exclude patient #2 who died before the time period]
  - Prevalence: (7/9)
  - Type of prevalence: (period prevalence)
- **Incidence of lung cancer from 1/1/2016–1/1/2017**
  - Number of patients who developed lung cancer in this time period: (4)
  - Number of patients at risk in this time period: (6) [exclude patients who were already sick at the start of the time period and those who died before the time period]
  - Incidence: (4/6)

Crude, Specific, and Standardized Rates

Crude rate is the actual measured rate for a **whole population**, e.g., rate of myocardial infarction for a whole population. Use caution using the crude rate, though. Imagine that in a given city, there are a lot of older, retired people—the crude rate of myocardial infarction will appear higher even though the rate for each age group has not actually changed.

Specific rate is the actual measured rate for **subgroup of population**, e.g., "age-specific" or "sex-specific" rate, e.g., the rate of myocardial infarction among people age >65 in the population, or the rate of breast cancer among the female population.

If you are provided specific rates, you can calculate the crude rate. The crude rate of an entire population is a weighted sum of each of the specific rates. The weighted specific rates that are added together is calculated in the table below.

Standardized rate (or adjusted rate) is adjusted to make groups equal on some factor, e.g., age; an "as if" statistic for comparing groups. The standardized rate adjusts or removes any difference between two populations based on the standardized variable. This allows an "uncontaminated" or unconfounded comparison.

Table 1-2. Types of Mortality Rate

Crude mortality rate	$\frac{\text{Deaths}}{\text{Population}}$	Deaths in a city in 2016 per population of the city	Crude rate of people dying in the population
Cause-specific mortality rate	$\frac{\text{Deaths from cause}}{\text{Population}}$	Deaths from lung cancer in a city in 2016 per population of the city	Specific rate of people dying from a particular disease in the population
Case-fatality rate	$\frac{\text{Deaths from cause}}{\text{Number of persons with the disease/cause}}$	Deaths from Ebola in a city per number of persons with Ebola	How likely you are to die from the disease,i.e., fatality
Proportionate mortality rate (PMR)	$\frac{\text{Deaths from cause}}{\text{All deaths}}$	Deaths from diabetes mellitus in a city per total deaths in the city	How much a disease contributes to the mortality rate, i.e., what proportion of the mortality rate is due to that disease

For example, the city of Hoboken, New Jersey has a population of 50,000. In 2016, the total number of deaths in Hoboken was 400. The number of deaths from lung cancer in Hoboken was 10, while the number of patients with lung cancer diagnosis was 30. Calculate the following:

- Mortality rate in Hoboken for 2016: (400/50,000 × 1,000)
- Cause specific mortality rate for lung cancer in Hoboken for 2016: (10/50,000 × 100,000)
- CFR for lung cancer in Hoboken in 2016: (10/30 × 100)
- PMR for lung cancer in Hoboken in 2016: (10/400 × 100)

PREVENTION

The goals of prevention in medicine are to **promote health**, **preserve health**, **restore health when it is impaired**, and **minimize suffering and distress**. These goals aim to minimize both morbidity and mortality.

- **Primary prevention** promotes health at both individual and community levels by facilitating health-enhancing behaviors, preventing the onset of risk behaviors, and diminishing exposure to environmental hazards. **Primary prevention efforts decrease disease incidence**. Examples include implementation of exercise programs and healthy food programs in schools.
- **Secondary prevention** screens for risk factors and early detection of asymptomatic or mild disease, permitting timely and effective intervention and curative treatment. **Secondary prevention efforts decrease disease prevalence**. Examples include recommended annual colonoscopy for patients age >65 and HIV testing for health care workers with needlestick injuries.
- **Tertiary prevention** reduces long-term impairments and disabilities and prevents repeated episodes of clinical illness. **Tertiary prevention efforts prevent recurrence and slow progression.** Examples include physical therapy for spinal injury patients and daily low-dose aspirin for those with previous myocardial infarction.

Consider a new healthcare bill that is being funded to help wounded war veterans gain access to prosthetic limb replacement. That would be considered tertiary prevention. The patients who would have access to the service have already been injured. The prosthetic devices would help reduce complications of amputation and help their rehabilitation. By improving quality of life and reducing morbidity, that is an implementation of tertiary prevention.

Now consider a medical student who is asked to wear a nose and mouth mask before entering the room of a patient with meningococcal meningitis. That would be considered primary prevention. Because the bacteria in this case can be spread by respiratory contact, the use of the mask will prevent the student from being exposed.

SCREENING TESTS

Screening tests help physicians to detect the presence of disease, e.g., an ELISA test for HIV, the results of which are either positive or negative for disease. The efficacy of a screening test is assessed by comparing the results to verified sick and healthy populations. For HIV, we would use a Western blot as a gold-standard.

The qualifier "true" or "false" is used to describe the correlation between the test results (positive or negative) and the disease (presence or absence).

True-positive (TP): tested positive, actually sick

- In other words, the positive result is true.

False-positive (FP): tested positive, is actually healthy

- In other words, the positive result is false.

True-negative (TN): tested negative, actually healthy

- In other words, the negative result is true.

False-negative (FN): tested negative, is actually sick

- In other words, the negative result is false.

Table 1-3. Screening Results in a 2 × 2 Table

		Disease				
		Present		Absent		Totals
Screening Test Results	Positive	TP	60	FP	70	TP + FP
	Negative	FN	40	TN	30	TN + FN
	Totals	TP + FN		TN + FP		TP + TN + FP + FN

Measures of Test Performance

Sensitivity and **specificity** are measures of the test performance (and in some cases, physical findings and symptoms). They help to provide additional information in cases where it is not possible to use a gold-standard test and instead a cheaper and easier (yet imperfect) screening test is used. Think about what would happen if you called the cardiology fellow to do a cardiac catheterization (the gold standard test to diagnose acute myocardial ischemia) on a patient without first having an EKG.

Sensitivity is the probability of correctly identifying a case of disease. In other words, it is the **proportion of truly diseased persons** in the screened population who are **identified as diseased** by the screening test. This is also known as the "true positive rate."

Sensitivity = TP/(TP + FN) = true positives/(true positives + false negatives)

- Measures only the distribution of persons with disease
- Uses data from the left column of the 2 × 2 table
- Note: 1-sensitivity = false negative rate

Note

A mnemonic for the clinical use of sensitivity is **SN-N-OUT** (sensitive test-negative-rules out disease).

If a test has a **high sensitivity**, then a **negative result** indicates the **absence of the disease.** For example, temporal arteritis (TA), a large vessel vasculitis that involves branches of the external carotid artery seen in those age >50, always shows elevated ESR. So 100% of patients with TA have elevated ESR. The sensitivity of an abnormal ESR for TA is 100%. If a patient you suspect of having TA has a normal ESR, then the patient does not have TA.

If there are 200 sick people, the sensitivity of a test tells us the capacity of the test to correctly identify these sick people. If a screening test identifies 160 of them as sick (they test positive), then the sensitivity of the test is 160/200 = 80%.

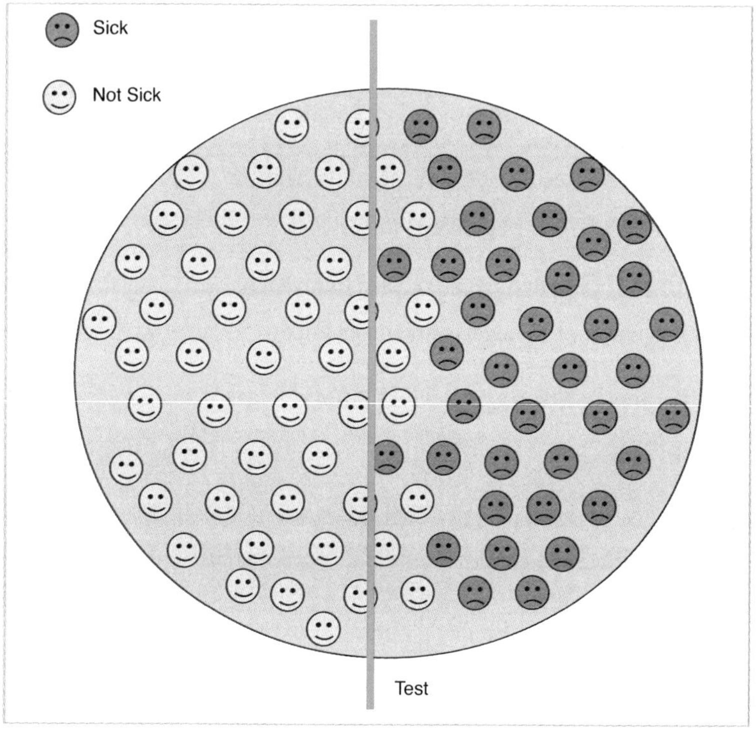

Figure 1-6. Sensitive Test

Specificity is the probability of correctly identifying disease-free persons. Specificity is the **proportion of truly nondiseased persons** who are **identified as nondiseased** by the screening test. This is also known as the "true negative rate."

Specificity = TN/(TN + FP) = true negatives/(true negatives + false positives)

- Measures only the distribution of persons who are disease-free
- Uses data from the right column of the 2 × 2 table
- Note: 1-specificity = false positive rate

If a test has a **high specificity**, then a **positive result** indicates the **existence of the disease.** For example, CT angiogram has a very high specificity for pulmonary embolism (97%). A CT scan read as positive for pulmonary embolism is likely true.

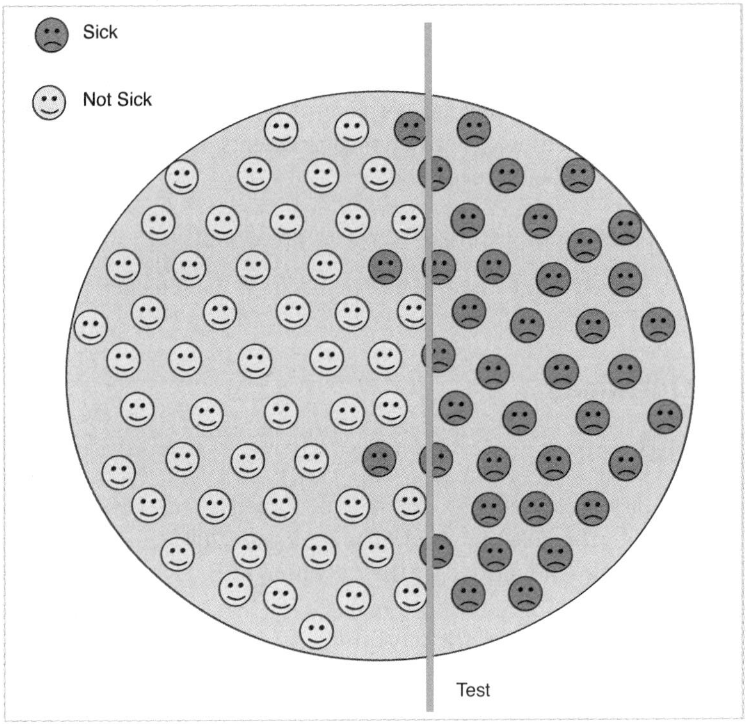

Figure 1-7. Specific Test

The separation between the sick and healthy in a given population isn't always clear; there is a measure of overlap, as in the figure above. In order to create a test that is specific and identifies only sick people as positive, it must (a) correctly identify all the healthy people and (b) not inaccurately identify healthy people as sick. In other words, the more specific the test, the fewer false-positives (i.e., healthy people incorrectly identified as sick) it will have. Specificity is therefore the capacity of a test to correctly exclude healthy people with negative test results.

Post-Test Probabilities

Positive predictive value (PPV) is the probability of disease in a person who receives a positive test result. The probability that a **person with a positive test is a true positive.** (i.e., has the disease) is referred to as the "predictive value of a positive test."

$$\textbf{PPV} = TP/(TP + FP)$$
$$= \text{true positives}/(\text{true positives} + \text{false positives})$$

PPV measures only the distribution of persons who receive a positive test result.

Negative predictive value (NPV) is the probability of no disease in a person who receives a negative test result. The probability that a **person with a negative test is a true negative** (i.e., does not have the disease) is referred to as the "predictive value of a negative test."

$$\text{NPV} = TN/(TN + FN)$$
$$= \text{true negatives}/(\text{true negatives} + \text{false negatives})$$

Note

A mnemonic for the clinical use of specificity: **SP-I-N** (specific test-positive-rules in disease).

Note

For any test, there is usually a trade-off between SNNOUT and SPIN. The trade-off can be represented graphically as the screening dimension curves and ROC curves.

NPV measures only the distribution of persons who receive a negative test result.

Accuracy is the total percentage correctly selected, the degree to which a measurement, or an estimate based on measurements, represents the true value of the attribute that is being measured.

$$\begin{aligned}\text{Accuracy} &= (\text{TP} + \text{TN})/(\text{TP} + \text{TN} + \text{FP} + \text{FN}) \\ &= (\text{true positives} + \text{true negatives})/\text{total screened patients}\end{aligned}$$

Review Questions

<u>Questions 1–3</u>

A screening test identifies 150 out of 1,000 patients to have tuberculosis. When tested with the gold standard diagnostic test, 200 patients test positive, including 100 of those identified by the screening test.

1. What is the sensitivity of the screening test?

2. What is the specificity of the screening test?

3. What is the positive predictive value?

Answers and Explanations

1. **Answer: 50%.** Sensitivity would be true positives divided by all sick people. Only 100 of the 150 positive results were actually true, so true positives would be 100. Total sick people is 200. So we have 100/200, making sensitivity 50%.

2. **Answer: 93.75%.** Specificity would be true negatives divided by all healthy people. Only 100 of the 150 positive results were actually true, so false positives (healthy people with a positive result) would be 50. Total people is 1000. So we have 1000 − 200 sick, making 800 healthy. True negatives = 800 − 50 so 750. Specificity = 750/800 so 93.75%.

3. **Answer: 66%.** Positive predictive value is true positives divided by all positives. Only 100 of the 150 positive results were actually true, so true positives would be 100. The total who tested positive would be 150. Therefore, PPV is 100 divided by 150 so 66%.

Effective Prevalence

Prevalence, which is a quantified measure of disease or cases in the population, is a relevant pre-test probability of disease within the population. The **more disease in a population, i.e., high prevalence**, the greater the probability that a positive test represents actual disease (= greater PPV). The **less disease in a population, i.e., lower prevalence**, the higher the probability that a negative result is true (= greater negative predictive value).

Consider this example: Among 80-year-old diabetic patients, the prevalence of kidney failure is higher than in the general population. This increased prevalence makes a physician more likely to believe the results of a screening test that shows kidney failure for an 80-year-old diabetic patient. We intuitively understand that the PPV is higher because this cohort of patients has a higher prevalence of disease.

Conversely, if a 15-year-old girl tests positive for a myocardial infarction, a physician will find the results strange and will thus repeat the test to confirm the positive result is not a false-positive. That is because the prevalence of myocardial infarction among teenage girls is so low that a positive result is more likely to be a mistake than a case of an actual myocardial infarction. In a teenage girl, a negative result for myocardial infarction is more likely to be true (high negative predictive value) because there is a very low prevalence of disease in this age group population.

Incidence is a measure of new cases in a population. Increasing the incidence would have no effect on sensitivity or PPV because a screening test can only detect the current presence or absence of disease, not its onset.

Prevalence has no effect on the sensitivity or specificity of a test. Those are metrics of the test and can be changed only by changing the test itself.

Double Hump Graph

In the graph below, which cutoff point provides optimal sensitivity?

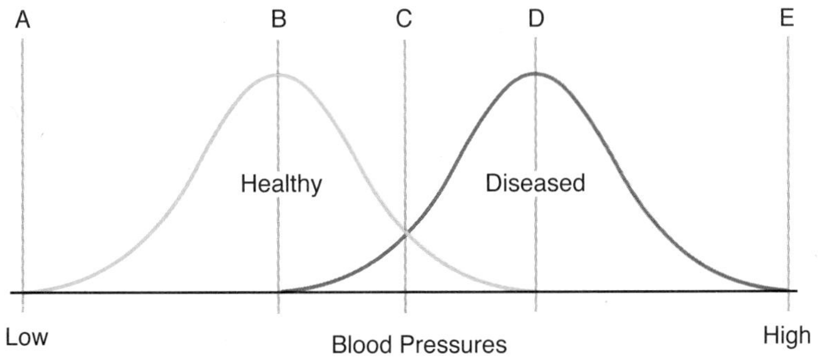

Figure 1-8. Healthy and Diseased Populations Along a Screening Dimension

Cutoff point B correctly identifies all the sick patients. It has the highest sensitivity (identifies all the sick patients). Cutoff D would be the most specific test (it identifies only sick people). Cutoff C where the 2 curves intersect is the most accurate. Note, the point of optimum sensitivity equals the point of optimum negative predictive value, while the point of optimum specificity equals the point of optimum positive predictive value.

Consider another example. Which of the following curves indicates the best screening test?

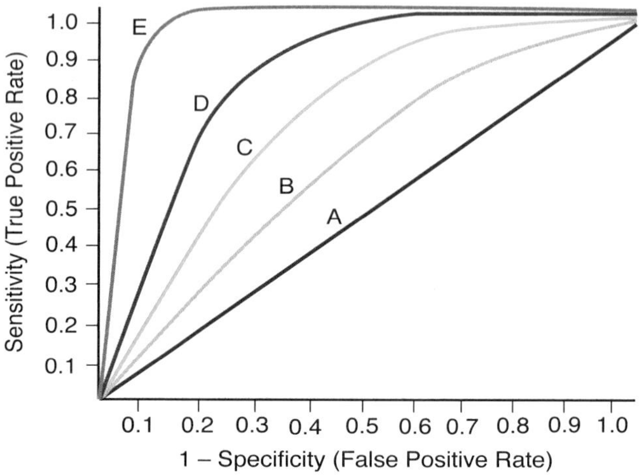

Figure 1-9. Receiver Operating Characteristic (ROC) Curves

Curve E achieves the highest sensitivity (y-axis) without including too many false-positives (x-axis).

STUDY DESIGNS

Bias in Research

Bias in research is a deviation from the truth of inferred results. It can be done intentionally or unintentionally.

Reliability is the ability of a test to **measure something consistently**, either across testing situations (test-retest reliability), within a test (split-half reliability), or across judges (inter-rater reliability). Think of the clustering of rifle shots at a target (precision).

Validity is the degree to which a test **measures that which was intended**. Think of a marksman hitting the bull's-eye. Reliability is a necessary, but insufficient, condition for validity (accuracy).

Types of bias

When there is **selection bias** (sampling bias), the sample selected is **not representative** of the population. Examples:

- Predicting rates of heart disease by gathering subjects from a local health club
- Using only hospital records to estimate population prevalence (Berkson bias)
- Including people in a study who are different from those who are not included (nonrespondent bias)
- **Solution**: random, independent sample; weight data

When there is **measurement bias**, information is gathered in a manner that **distorts the information**. Examples:

- Measuring patient satisfaction with their physicians by using leading questions, e.g., "You don't like your doctor, do you?"
- Subjects' behavior is altered because they are being studied; this is only a factor when there is no control group in a prospective study (Hawthorne effect)
- **Solution**: have a control group

When there is **experimenter expectancy** (Pygmalion effect), **experimenters' expectations are inadvertently communicated** to subjects, who then produce the desired effects. **Solution**: use **double-blind** design, where neither the subject nor the investigators know which group receives the intervention.

Lead-time bias gives a **false estimate of survival rates**, e.g., patients seem to live longer with the disease after it is uncovered by a screening test. Actually, there is no increased survival, but because the disease is discovered sooner, patients who are diagnosed *seem* to live longer. **Solution**: use life-expectancy to assess benefit.

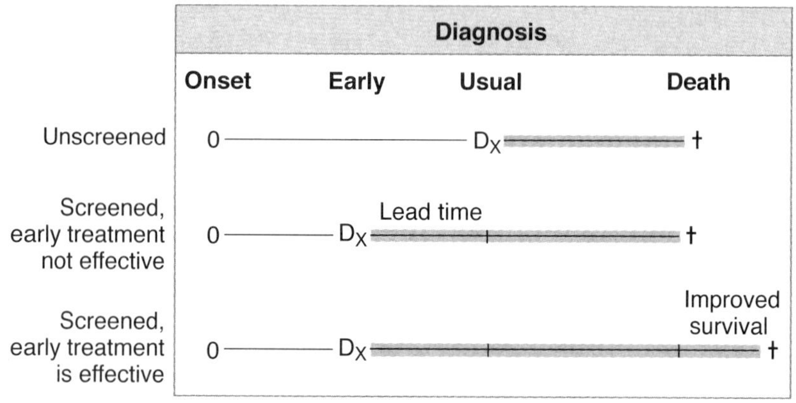

Figure 1-8. Diagnosis, Time, and Survival

When there is **recall bias**, subjects **fail to accurately recall events** in the past. For example: "How many times last year did you kiss your mother?" This is a likely problem in retrospective studies. **Solution**: confirmation.

When there is **late-look bias**, individuals with **severe disease are less likely to be uncovered** in a survey **because they die first**. For example, a recent survey found that persons with AIDS reported only mild symptoms. **Solution**: stratify by disease severity.

When there is **confounding bias**, the factor being examined **is related to other factors of less interest**. Unanticipated factors obscure a relationship or make it seem like there is one when there is not. More than one explanation can be found for the presented results. For example, compare the relationship between exercise and heart disease in 2 populations when one population is younger and the other is older. Are differences in heart disease due to exercise or to age? **Solution**: combine the results from multiple studies, meta-analysis.

When there is **design bias**, parts of the study **do not fit together** to answer the question of interest. The most common issue is a non-comparable control group. For example, compare the effects of an anti-hypertensive drug in hypertensives versus normotensives. **Solution**: random assignment, i.e., subjects assigned to treatment or control group by a random process.

Table 1-4. Type of Bias in Research

Type of Bias	Definition	Important Associations	Solutions
Selection	Sample not representative	Berkson's bias, nonrespondent bias	Random, independent sample
Measurement	Gathering the information distorts it	Hawthorne effect	Control group/placebo group
Experimenter expectancy	Researcher's beliefs affect outcome	Pygmalion effect	Double-blind design
Lead-time	Early detection confused with increased survival	Benefits of screening	Measure "back-end" survival
Recall	Subjects cannot remember accurately	Retrospective studies	Multiple sources to confirm information

Type of Bias	Definition	Important Associations	Solutions
Late-look	Severely diseased individuals are not uncovered	Early mortality	Stratify by severity
Confounding	Unanticipated factors obscure results	Hidden factors affect results	Multiple studies, good research design
Design	Parts of study do not fit together	Non-comparable control group	Random assignment

TYPES OF RESEARCH STUDIES

Observational Study

In an observational study, nature is allowed to take its course, i.e., there is no intervention.

- **Case report:** brief, objective report of a clinical characteristic/outcome from a single clinical subject or event, $n = 1$, e.g., 23-year-old man with treatment-resistant TB; there is no control group
- **Case series report:** objective report of a clinical characteristic/outcome from a group of clinical subjects, $n > 1$, e.g., patients at local hospital with treatment-resistant TB; there is no control group
- **Cross-sectional study:** the presence or absence of disease (and other variables) are determined in each member of the study population or representative sample at a particular time; co-occurrence of a variable and the disease can be examined
  - Disease prevalence, not incidence, is recorded
  - Cannot usually determine temporal sequence of cause and effect, e.g., who in the community now has treatment-resistant TB
- **Case-control study:** a group of people with the disease is identified and compared with a suitable comparison group without the disease; almost always retrospective, e.g., compares cases of treatment-resistant TB with those of nonresistant TB
  - Cannot usually assess incidence or prevalence of disease, but it can help determine causal relationships
  - Very useful for studying conditions with very low incidence or prevalence
- **Cohort study:** population group of those who have been **exposed to risk factor** is identified and followed over time and **compared with a group not exposed to the risk factor**. Outcome is disease incidence in each group, e.g., following a prison inmate population and marking the development of treatment-resistant TB
  - Prospective, meaning that subjects are tracked forward in time
  - Can determine incidence and causal relationships, and must follow population long enough for incidence to appear.

Note

- Random error is unfortunate but okay and expected (a threat to reliability).
- Systematic error is bad and biases result (a threat to validity).

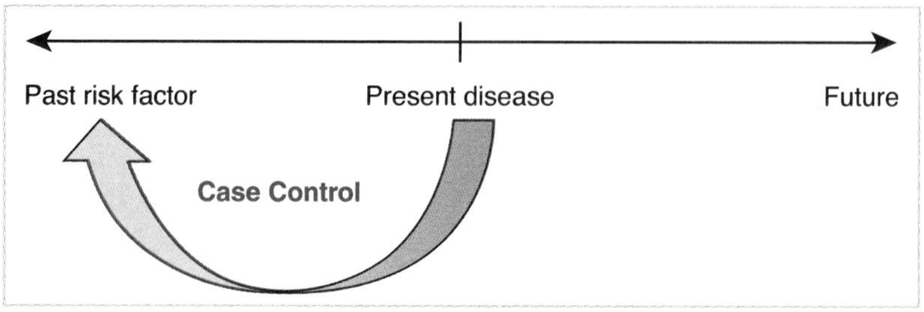

Figure 1-9. Retrospective Study

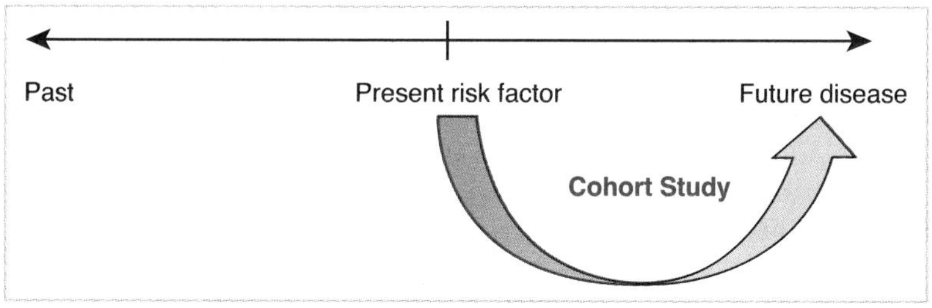

Figure 1-10. Prospective Study

Cohort Study		
Risk Factor	**Disease**	**No Disease**
	60 A	240 B
No Risk Factor	60 C	540 D

Cohort Study

Relative risk (RR) is a comparative probability asking, "How much more likely?" To find it, calculate the IR of the **exposed group divided by** the IR of the **unexposed group**. How much greater chance does one group have of contracting the disease compared with the other group?

Attributable risk (AR) is a comparative probability asking "How many more cases in one group?" To find it, calculate the IR of **exposed group minus** the IR of the **unexposed group**.

Note: Both relative and attributable risk tell us if there are differences, but they do not tell us why those differences exist.

Interpretation: for every 100 people treated, 1 case will be prevented.

Let's first consider **RR**. If we compare a group of 100 children who live near a chemical plant (risk factor) to a group of 100 children who do not (no risk factor), and follow them over time to see who develops asthma, we can calculate how much more likely it is for those exposed to the risk factor to develop disease, i.e., RR. In this example, say 20 children near the chemical plant and 5 children not living near the plant all develop asthma.

$$RR = \frac{\text{Incidence in exposed group (risk factor)}}{\text{Incidence in unexposed group (no risk factor)}}$$

$$= \frac{20}{100} \div \frac{5}{100} = 4$$

Interpretation: a child living near the chemical plant is 4x more likely to develop asthma than a child not living near the plant

Now let's consider **AR**. Are all 20 cases among those living near the plant due to the proximity of the plant? We know that 5 children developed asthma even though they did not live next to plant, meaning that some of the 20 cases are not necessarily due to the risk factor itself (in this case, the chemical plant).

How many of the 20 cases are due to the risk factor or, in other words, are attributable to the risk factor?

AR = Incidence in exposed group – Incidence in unexposed group

$$\frac{20}{100} - \frac{5}{100} = \frac{15}{100}$$

Interpretation: for every 100 children exposed to the risk factor, 15 cases are attributable to the risk factor itself; in other words, when we expose 100 children, 15 cases of asthma will be caused by the exposure.

So what is the **NNH**? NNH is the inverse of the attributable risk.

$$= \frac{100}{15} = 6.66 = 7 \text{ (always round up)}$$

Interpretation: for every 7 people exposed to the risk factor, there will be 1 case.

Case Control Study

For a case-control study, use **odds ratio (OR)**, which looks at the increased odds of getting a disease with exposure to a risk factor versus nonexposure to that factor. Find the odds of **exposure for cases divided by** odds of **exposure for controls**, for example: the odds that a person with lung cancer was a smoker versus the odds that a person without lung cancer was a smoker.

Table 1-5. Case-Control Study: Lung Cancer and Smoking

	Lung Cancer	No Lung Cancer
Smokers	659 (A)	984 (B)
Nonsmokers	25 (C)	348 (D)

$$\text{Odds ratio} = \frac{A/C}{B/D} = \frac{AD}{BC}$$

Use OR = AD/BC as the working formula. For the above example:

$$OR = \frac{AD}{BC} = \frac{659 \times 348}{984 \times 25} = 9.32$$

Interpretation: the odds of having been a smoker are over 9x greater for someone with lung cancer compared with someone without lung cancer.

Odds ratio does not so much predict disease as it does estimate the strength of a risk factor.

How would you analyze the data from the following case-control study?

Case-Control Study: Colorectal Cancer and Family History

	No Colorectal Cancer	Colorectal Cancer	TOTALS
Family History of Colorectal Cancer	120	60	180
No Family History of Colorectal Cancer	200	20	220
TOTALS	320	80	400
ANSWER:	$\frac{AD}{BC}$	$\frac{(60)(200)}{(120)(20)}$	OR = 5.0

Interpretation: the odds of having a family history of colorectal cancer are 5x greater for those who have the disease than for those who do not.

Table 1-6. Differentiating Observational Studies

Characteristic	Cross-Sectional Studies	Case-Control Studies	Cohort Studies
Time	One time point	Retrospective	Prospective
Incidence	NO	NO	YES
Prevalence	YES	NO	NO
Causality	NO	YES	YES
Role of disease	Prevalence of disease	Begin with disease	End with disease
Assesses	Association of risk factor and disease	Many risk factors for single disease	Single risk factor affecting many diseases
Data analysis	*Chi*-square to assess association	Odds ratio to estimate risk	Relative risk to estimate risk

Clinical Trials

Researchers design clinical trials to answer specific research questions related to a medical product. A **control group** (often the *placebo* group) will includes subjects who **do not receive the intervention under study**, used as a **source of comparison** to be certain the experiment group is being affected by the intervention and not by other factors. Control group subjects must be **as similar as possible to intervention group** subjects.

For a medical product to receive approval by the Food and Drug Administration (FDA), 3 phases must be passed.

- **Phase 1**: testing safety in healthy volunteers
- **Phase 2**: testing protocol and dose levels in a small group of patient volunteers
- **Phase 3** (**definitive test**): testing efficacy and occurrence of side effects in a larger group of patient volunteers

Post-FDA approval, marketing surveys will collect reports of drug side effects among populations commonly using the product.

In a **randomized controlled clinical trial (RCT)**, subjects are **randomly allocated** into "intervention" and "control" groups to receive or not receive an experimental/preventive/therapeutic procedure or intervention. This is generally regarded as the **most scientifically rigorous** type of study available in epidemiology.

A **double-blind RCT** is the type of study **least subject to bias**, but also the **most expensive** to conduct. Double-blind means that neither subjects nor researchers know whether the subjects are in the treatment or comparison group. A double-blind study has 2 types of control groups:

- Placebos (25–40% often show improvement in placebo group)
- Standard of care (current treatment versus new treatment)

A **community trial** is an experiment in which the unit of allocation to receive a preventive or therapeutic regimen is an **entire community or political subdivision**. Does the treatment work in real-world circumstances?

A **cross-over study** is one in which, for ethical reasons, no group involved can remain untreated. **All subjects receive the intervention** but at different times (making recruitment of subjects easier). Assume double-blind design. For example, an AZT trial, where group A receives AZT for 3 months while group B is the control. For the second 3 months, group B receives AZT and group A is the control.

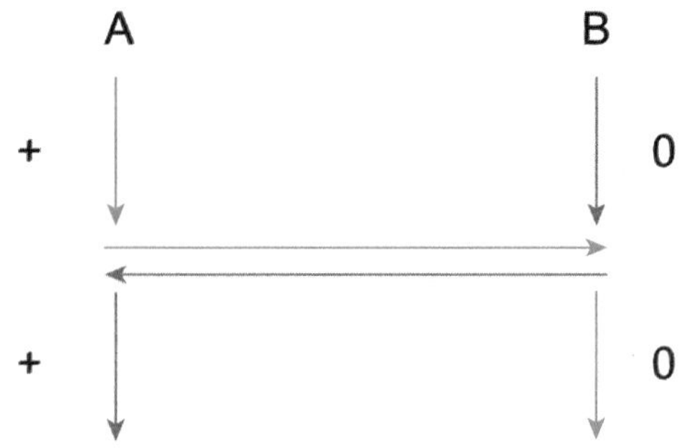

Figure 1-11. Cross-Over Study

Biostatistics 2

Learning Objectives

- ❑ Demonstrate understanding of key probability rules
- ❑ Summarize data
- ❑ Solve problems using inferential statistics
- ❑ Use knowledge of nominal, ordinal, interval, and ratio scales
- ❑ Answer questions about statistical tests

KEY PROBABILITY RULES

Independent Events

Events are **independent** if the **occurrence of one tells you nothing about the occurrence of the other**. Combine probabilities for independent events by **multiplication**.

The issue here is the intersection of 2 sets; e.g., if the chance of having blond hair is 0.3 and the chance of having a cold is 0.2, the chance of meeting a blond-haired person with a cold is: $0.3 \times 0.2 = 0.06$ (or 6%).

If events are **nonindependent**, multiply the probability of one event by the probability of the second, assuming that the first has occurred; e.g., if a box has 5 white balls and 5 black balls, the chance of picking 2 black balls is:

$$\frac{5}{10} \times \frac{4}{9} = 0.5 \times 0.44 = 0.22 \text{ (or 22\%)}$$

Mutually Exclusive Events

Events are mutually exclusive if the **occurrence of one event precludes the occurrence of the other**. Combine probabilities for mutually exclusive outcomes by **addition**.

The issue here is the union of two sets; e.g., if a coin lands on heads, it cannot be tails; the events are **mutually exclusive**. If a coin is flipped, the chance that it will be either heads or tails is $0.5 + 0.5 = 1.0$ (or 100%)

If 2 events are **not mutually exclusive**, add them together and subtract out the multiplied probabilities to get the combination of probabilities. For example, if the chance of having diabetes is 10% and the chance of being obese is 30%, the chance of meeting someone who is obese or has diabetes or both is $0.1 + 0.3 - (0.1 \times 0.3) = 0.37$ (or 37%).

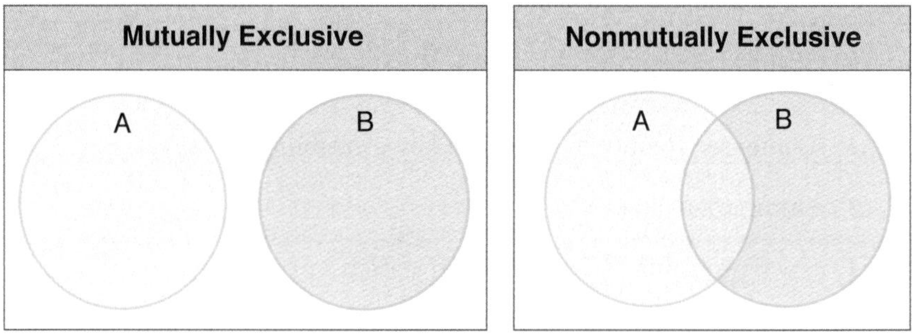

Figure 2-1. Venn Diagram of Mutually Exclusive and Nonmutually Exclusive Events

Review Questions

1. If the prevalence of diabetes is 10%, what is the chance that 3 people selected at random from the population will all have diabetes?

2. Chicago has a population of 10,000,000. If 25% of the population is Latino, 30% is African American, 5% is Arab American, and 40% is of European extraction, how many people in Chicago are classified as other than of European extraction?

3. At age 65, the probability of surviving for the next 5 years is 0.8 for a white man and 0.9 for a white woman. For a married couple who are both white and age 65, the probability that the wife will be a living widow 5 years later is:

   A. 90%

   B. 72%

   C. 18%

   D. 10%

   E. 8%

4. If the chance of surviving for 1 year after being diagnosed with prostate cancer is 80% and the chance of surviving for 2 years after diagnosis is 60%, what is the chance of surviving for 2 years after diagnosis, given that the patient is alive at the end of the first year?

   A. 20%

   B. 48%

   C. 60%

   D. 75%

   E. 80%

Answers and Explanations

1. **Answer: 0.001.** 0.1 × 0.1 × 0.1 = 0.001

2. **Answer: 6,000,000.** 25% + 30% + 5% = 60%. 60% × 10,000,000 = 6,000,000

3. **Answer: C.** You're being asked for the joint probability of independent events; therefore, the probabilities are multiplied. Chance of the wife being alive: 90%, and chance of the husband being dead: 100% – 80% = 20%. Therefore, 0.9 × 0.2 = 18%.

4. **Answer: D.** The question tests knowledge of "conditional probability." Out of 100 patients, 80 are alive at the end of 1 year and 60 at the end of 2 years. The 60 patients alive after 2 years are a subset of those that make it to the first year. Therefore, 60/80 = 75%.

DESCRIPTIVE STATISTICS

Distributions

Statistics deals with the world as distributions. These distributions are summarized by a **central tendency** and **variation around that center**. The most important distribution is the **normal** or **Gaussian curve**. This "bell-shaped" curve is **symmetric**, with one side the mirror image of the other.

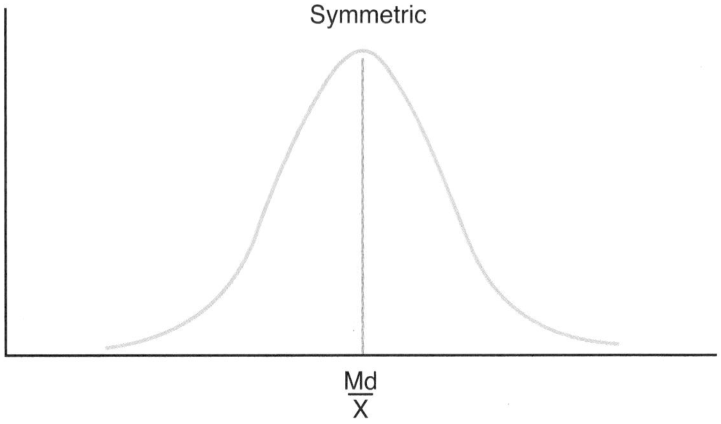

Figure 2-2. Measures of Central Tendency

Measures of central tendency

Central tendency describes a single value which attempts to describe a set of data by identifying the central (or middle) value within that set. (Colloquially, measures of central tendency are often called *averages*.) There are several valid measures:

- **Mean ($\overline{X}$)** (or *average*): sum of the values of the observations divided by the numbers of observations
- **Median (Md)**: point on the scale which divides a group into 2 parts (upper and lower half); the measurement below which half the observations fall is *50th percentile*
- **Mode**: **most frequently occurring value** in a set of observations

Given the distribution of numbers: 3, 6, 7, 7, 9, 10, 12, 15, 16, the **mode is 7**, the **median is 9**, and the **mean is 9.4**.

Not all curves are normal; sometimes the curve is **skewed** positively or negatively.

- A **positive skew** has the tail to the right, and the mean greater than the median.
- A **negative skew** has the tail to the left, and the median greater than the mean.

For skewed distributions, the **median** is a better representation of central tendency than is the mean.

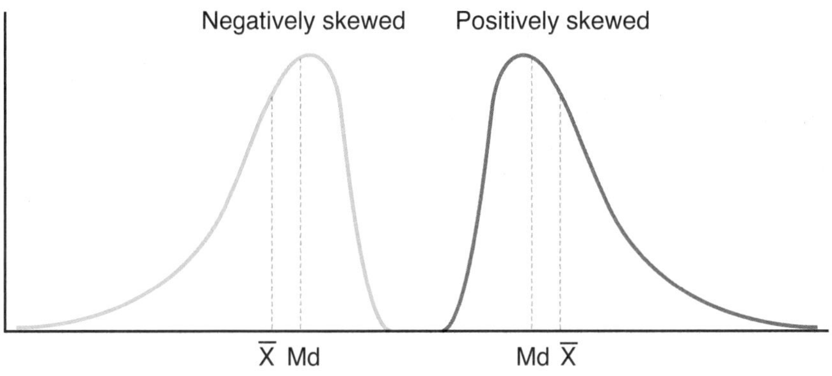

Figure 2-3. Skewed Distribution Curves

Measures of variability

The simplest measure of variability in statistics is the **range**, the difference between the highest and the lowest score. However, the range is unstable and can change easily. A more stable and more useful measure of dispersion is the **standard deviation (S** or **SD)**. To calculate the SD:

- First subtract the mean from each score to obtain **deviations from the mean**. This will give us both positive and negative values.
- Then square the deviations to make them all positive.
- Add the squared deviations together and divide by the number of cases.
- Take the square root of this average, and the result is the SD:

$$s = \sqrt{\frac{\Sigma\left(X - \bar{X}\right)^2}{n-1}}$$

The square of the SD (s^2) equals the **variance**.

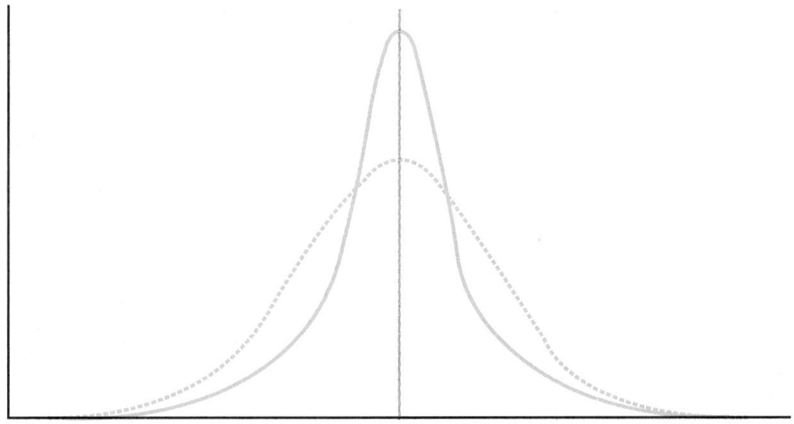

Figure 2-4. Two Normal Curves with the Same Mean but Different SD

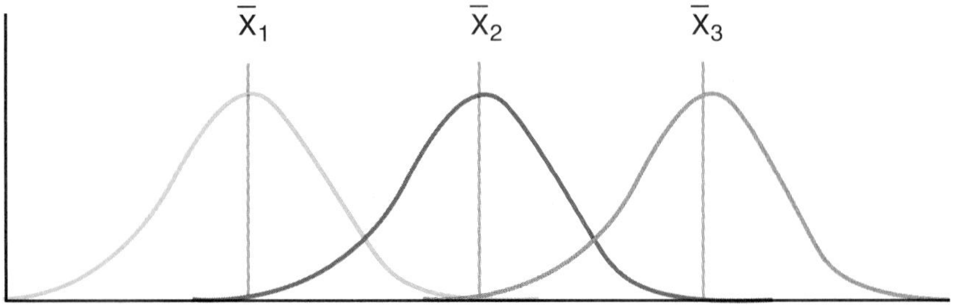

Figure 2-5. Three Normal Curves with Same SD but Different Mean

Note

On the exam you will not be asked to calculate SD and variance, but you will need to understand how they relate to the normal curve. Also, be able to combine the given SD constants to answer basic questions.

In any normal curve, a constant proportion of the cases fall within 1, 2, and 3 SDs of the mean: within 1 SD 68%; within 2 SDs 95.5%; and within 3 SDs 99.7%.

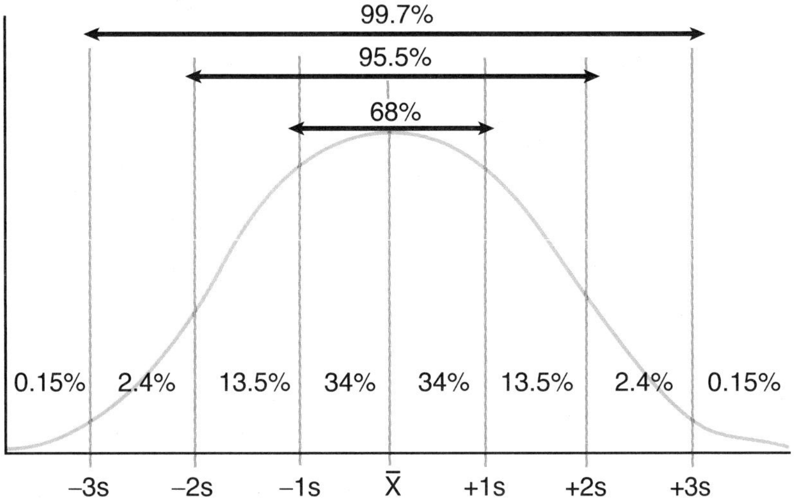

Figure 2-6. Percentage of Cases within 1, 2, and 3 SDs of the Mean in a Normal Distribution

Review Questions

5. In a normal distribution curve, what percent of the cases are below 2s below the mean?
6. In a normal distribution curve, what percent of the cases are above 1s below the mean?
7. A student who scores at the 97.5 percentile falls where on the curve?
8. A student took 2 tests: On test A his results were score 45%, mean 30%, and SD 5%. On test B the results were score 60%, mean 40%, and SD 10%. On which test did the student do better, relative to his classmates?

Answers and Explanations

5. **Answer:** 2.5%
6. **Answer:** 84%
7. **Answer:** 2 SD above the mean
8. **Answer:** On test A, he scored 3 SD above the mean versus only 2 SD above the mean for test B.

INFERENTIAL STATISTICS

The purpose of inferential statistics is to designate **how likely it is that a given finding is simply the result of chance**. Inferential statistics would not be necessary if investigators could study all members of a population. However, because that can rarely be done, using select samples that are representative of an entire population allows us to **generalize the results from the sample to the population**.

Confidence Interval

Confidence interval is a way of admitting that any measurement from a sample is only an **estimate** of the population, i.e., although the estimate given from the sample is likely to be close, the true values for the population may be above or below the sample values. A confidence interval **specifies how far above or below a sample-based value the population value lies** within a given range, from a possible high to a possible low. Reality, therefore, is most likely to be somewhere within the specified range.

To calculate the confidence interval: **study result +/– Z score × standard error**

Study result might be a mean, a relative risk or any other relevant measure that is the result of the data from the study itself. **Z score** depends on the level of confidence required. In medicine, the requirement is **at least a 95% confidence interval**. So the options are as follows:

- Z score for 95% confidence interval = 1.96 = 2
- Z score for 99% confidence interval = 2.58 = 2.5

While the SD measures the variability within a single sample, the **standard error** estimates the variability *between* samples. The standard error is usually provided. The smaller the standard error, the better and more precise the study. The standard error is affected by 2 factors: the SD and the sample size (n). The greater the SD, (high variation in the data), the greater the standard error, and the larger the sample size, the smaller the standard error.

$$\textbf{Standard Error} = \frac{SD}{\sqrt{n}}$$

Suppose 100 students in the 9th grade have just taken their final exam, and the mean score was 64% with SD 15. The 95% confidence interval of the mean for 9th grade students in the population would be as follows:

- Mean = 65
- Z score for 95% confidence = 2 (rounded up Z score)
- SD = 15
- Sample size = 100

$$\text{Plug in the numbers: Mean} +/- \text{Z score } \frac{SD}{\sqrt{n}}$$

$$\text{or } 65 +/- 2(15/10) = 65 +/- 3$$

What this means is that we are 95% sure that the mean score of 9th graders in the population will fall somewhere between 62 and 68.

Assuming the graph below presents 95% confidence intervals, which groups, if any, are statistically different from each other?

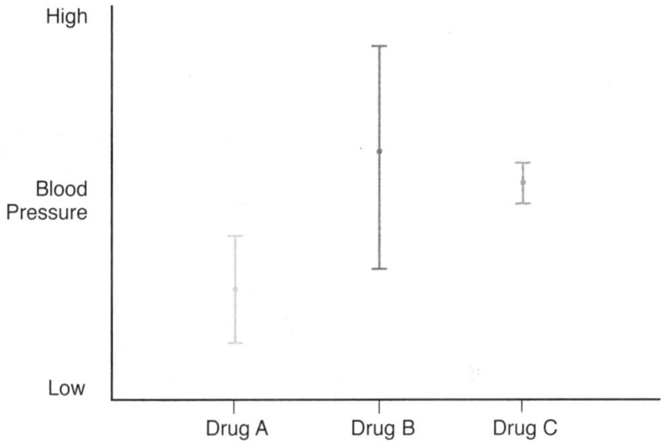

Blood Pressure at End of Clinical Trial for 3 Drugs

When comparing 2 groups, any overlap of confidence intervals means the groups are not significantly different. If the graph represents 95% confidence intervals, drugs B and C are no different in their effects; drug B is no different from drug A and drug A has a better effect than drug C.

For the confidence interval for **relative risk and odds ratios**, consider the following: **If the given confidence interval contains 1.0, then there is no statistically significant effect of exposure**. For example:

Relative Risk	Confidence Interval	Interpretation
1.77	(1.22 – 2.45)	Statistically significant (increased risk)
1.63	(0.85 – 2.46)	NOT statistically significant (risk is the same)
0.78	(0.56 – 0.94)	Statistically significant (decreased risk)

If **RR** >**1.0**, then subtract 1.0 and read as percent increase. So 1.77 means one group has 77% more cases than the other. If **RR** <**1.0**, then subtract from 1.0 and read as reduction in risk. So 0.78 means one group has a 22% reduction in risk.

Statistical Inference

The goal of science is to define reality. Think of statistics as the referee in the game of science. We have all agreed to play the game according to the judgment calls of the referee, even though we know the referee can, and will, be wrong at times. The basic steps of statistical inference are as follows:

1. Define the **research question**: what are you trying to show?
2. Define the **null hypothesis** (generally the opposite of what you hope to show). Null hypothesis says that the **findings are the result of**

chance or random factors. If you want to show that a drug works, the null hypothesis will be that the drug does NOT work. The **alternative hypothesis** says what is left after defining the null hypothesis. In this example, that the drug does actually work.

There are 2 types of null hypothesis:

- **One-tailed**, i.e., directional or "one-sided," such that one group is greater than or less than the other (Group A is not *less* than Group B, or Group A is not *greater than* Group B)
- **Two-tailed**, i.e., nondirectional or "two-sided," such that 2 groups are not the same (Group A $\neq$ Group B)

Once the data are collected and analyzed by the appropriate statistical test, the **hypothesis testing** is begun. How to run these tests is not tested on the exam, but you may need to be able to interpret results of statistical tests with which you are presented.

Note

We never accept the null hypothesis. We either reject it or fail to reject it. Saying we do not have sufficient evidence to reject it is not the same as being able to affirm that it is true.

To interpret output from a statistical test, focus on the ***p*-value**. The term *p*-value refers to 2 things. In its first sense, the *p*-value is a standard against which we compare our results. In the second sense, the *p*-value is a result of computation. The **computed *p*-value is compared with the *p*-value criterion to test statistical significance**. If the computed value is less than the criterion, we have achieved statistical significance. In general, the smaller the *p* the better.

The *p*-value criterion is traditionally set at $p \leq 0.05$. (Assume that these are the criteria if no other value is explicitly specified.) Using this standard:

- If $p \leq 0.05$, reject the null hypothesis (reached statistical significance).
- If $p > 0.05$, do not reject the null hypothesis (has not reached statistical significance).

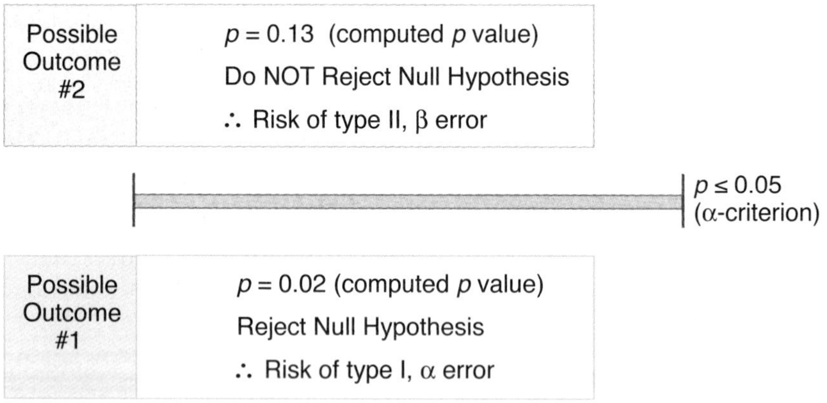

Figure 2-8. Making Decisions Using *p*-Values

- If $p = 0.02$, reject the null hypothesis, i.e., decide that the drug works.
- If $p = 0.13$, fail to reject the null hypothesis, i.e., decide that the drug does not work.

Types of error

If we do reject the null hypothesis, we are still not certain we are correct, i.e., the results given by the sample may be inconsistent with the full population. If that is true, any decision made on the basis of the sample could be in error.

Two types of errors can be made:

- **Type I error (α error): rejecting the null hypothesis when it is really true**
  - This type of error assumes a statistically significant effect on the basis of the sample when there is none in the population, e.g., asserting that the drug works when it doesn't.
  - The chance of type I error is given by the *p*-value; if $p = 0.05$, then the chance of a type I error is 5 in 100, or 1 in 20 if we reject the null hypothesis based on the evidence of the data.
- **Type II error (β error): failing to reject the null hypothesis when it is really false**
  - This type of error declares no significant effect on the basis of the sample when there really is one in the population, e.g., asserting the drug does not work when it really does.
  - The chance of a type II error cannot be directly estimated from the *p*-value.

The ***p*-value** here does a few things:

- Provides criterion for making decisions about the null hypothesis
- Quantifies the chance that a decision to reject the null hypothesis will be wrong
- Tells statistical significance, not clinical significance or likelihood of benefit

The *p*-value **does not** tell us:

- Chance that an individual patient will benefit
- Percentage of patients who will benefit
- Degree of benefit expected for a given patient

Statistical power

In statistics, **power** is the capacity to detect a difference if there is one. Just as increasing the power of a microscope makes it easier to see what is going on in histology, increasing statistical power allows us to detect what is happening in the data.

Power is directly related to type II error.

Power $= 1 - \beta$

There are several ways to increase statistical power. The most common is to increase sample size.

Note

A **type I error (error of commission)** is generally considered **worse** than a type II error (error of omission).

- If the null hypothesis is rejected, there is no chance of a type II error.
- If the null hypothesis is not rejected, there is no chance of a type I error.

		Reality	
		Drug Works	Drug Does Not Work
Research	Reject	Power	Type I Error
	Not Reject	Type II Error	

Note

For the exam, focus on **nominal** and **interval** scales.

SCALE

To convert the world into numbers, we use 4 types of scale: nominal, ordinal, interval, and ratio. Scales of measurement refer to ways in which numbers are categorized.

Table 2-1. Types of Scale in Statistics

Type of Scale	Description	Key Words	Examples
Nominal (Categorical)	Different groups	This or that	Gender, comparing among treatment interventions
Ordinal	Groups in sequence	Comparative quality, rank order	Olympic medals, class rank in medical school
Interval	Exact differences among groups	Quantity, mean, and standard deviation	Height, weight, blood pressure, drug dosage
Ratio	Interval + true zero point	Zero means zero	Temperature measured in degrees Kelvin

The scales as described below are hierarchically arranged, from **least information** provided (nominal) to **most information** provided (ratio). Any scale can be degraded to a lower scale, e.g., interval data can be treated as ordinal.

- **Nominal scale**
  - Puts people into categories without specifying the relationship between the categories
  - Example is gender, with 2 groups (male and female); other examples include drug versus control group
  - Anytime you can say, "It's either this or that," it is nominal scale
- **Ordinal scale** (or rank order)
  - Puts people into categories and specifies the relationship between them (quality)
  - What is not known is *how* different the categories are (quantity)
  - Example is saying Ben is taller than Fred; other examples include class rank in medical school and Olympic medals
- **Interval scale** (or numeric scale)
  - Uses a scale graded in equal increments
  - Allows us to say not only that 2 things are different, but also by *how much*

  - If a measurement has a mean and SD, treat it as an interval scale
  - Example is the scale of length: we know that 1 inch is equal to any other inch
- **Ratio scale (best measure)**
  - Orders things and contains equal intervals, but also has a **true zero point**
  - Zero is a floor, i.e., you can't go any lower
  - Example is measuring temperature using Kelvin scale

STATISTICAL TESTS

Selecting the correct statistical test for a research project will depend on the nature of the variables being studied.

Table 2-2. Types of Scale and Basic Statistical Tests

	Variables		
Name of Statistical Test	**Interval**	**Nominal**	**Comment**
Pearson correlation	2	0	Is there a linear relationship?
Chi-square	0	2	Any # of groups
t-test	1	1	2 groups only
One-way ANOVA	1	1	**2 or** more groups
Matched pairs *t*-test	1	1	2 groups, linked data pairs, before and after
Repeated measures ANOVA	1	1	More than 2 groups, linked data

ANOVA = Analysis of Variance

Correlation (r, −1.0 to +1.0)

Correlation, by itself, does not mean causation. A correlation coefficient indicates the degree to which 2 measures are related, not *why* they are related. In other words, it does not mean that one variable necessarily causes the other.

There are 2 types of correlation:

- **Pearson correlation**: compares 2 interval level variables
- **Spearman correlation**: compares 2 ordinal level variables

A **positive value** means that **2 variables go together in the same direction,** e.g., MCAT scores have a positive correlation with medical school grades.

A **negative value** means that the **presence of one variable is associated with the absence of another variable,** e.g., there is a negative correlation between age and quickness of reflexes.

The further from 0, the stronger the relationship ($r = 0$). A **zero correlation** means that **2 variables have no linear relation to one another,** e.g., height and success in medical school.

Note

Remember, your **default choices** are:

- Correlation for interval data
- *Chi*-square for nominal data
- *t*-test for a combination of nominal and interval data

Note

On the exam you will not be asked to compute statistical tests, but do recognize how and when they should be used.

You should, however, be able to interpret **scatterplots of data:** positive slope, negative slope, and which of a set of scatterplots indicates a stronger correlation.

Correlation can be graphed using a scatterplot, which shows points that approximate a line.

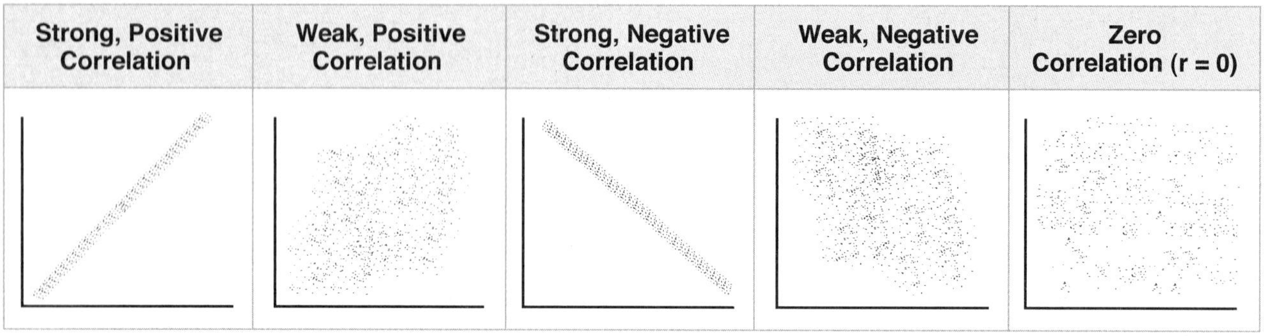

Figure 2-9. Scatterplots and Correlations

t-test

A *t*-test **compares the means of 2 groups** from a single nominal variable, using means from an interval variable to see whether the groups are different. The output of a *t*-test is a "*t*" statistic. It is used for 2 groups only, i.e., compares 2 means. For example, do patients with MI who are in psychotherapy have a reduced length of convalescence compared with those who are not in therapy?

- **Pooled** t-test is a regular t-test, assuming the variances of the 2 groups are the same
- **Matched pairs** t-test involves matching each person in one group with a person in second group; applies to before-and-after measures and linked data

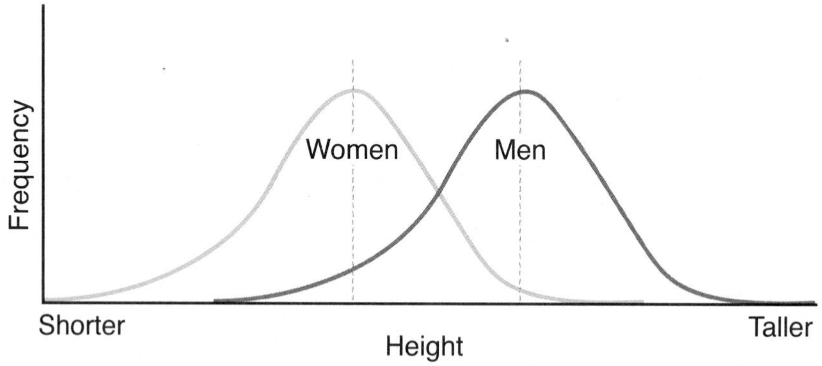

Figure 2-10. Comparison of the Distributions of 2 Groups

Analysis of Variance (ANOVA)

Output from an ANOVA is ≥1 F-statistics.

- **1-way ANOVA** compares means of many groups (≥2) of a single nominal variable using an interval variable. A significant p-value means that at least 2 of the tested groups are different.

- **2-way ANOVA** compares means of groups generated by 2 nominal variables using an interval variable. It can test the effects of several variables at the same time.
- **Repeated measures ANOVA** features multiple measurements of the same people over time.

Chi-square

A *chi*-square tests to see whether 2 nominal variables are independent, i.e., in order to test the efficacy of a new drug, compare the number of recovered patients given the drug with those who were not. *Chi*-square features nominal data only, and any number of groups (2×2, 2×3, 3×3, etc.).

Table 2-3. *Chi*-Square Analysis for Nominal Data

	New Drug	Placebo	Totals
Recovered	45	35	80
Not Recovered	15	25	40
Totals	60	60	120

Review Questions

9. A recent study finds a higher incidence of SIDS for children of mothers who smoke. If the rate for smoking mothers is 230/100,000 and the rate for nonsmoking mothers is 71/100,000, what is the relative risk for children of mothers who smoke?

   A. 159
   B. 32
   C. 230
   D. 3.2
   E. 8.4

10. A researcher wishing to demonstrate the efficacy of a new treatment for hypertension compares the effects of the new treatment versus a placebo. This study provides a test of the null hypothesis that the new treatment has no effect on hypertension. In this case, the null hypothesis should be considered as

    A. positive proof that the stated premise is correct
    B. the assertion of a statistically significant relationship
    C. the assumption that the study design is adequate
    D. the probability that the relationship being studied is the result of random factors
    E. the result the experimenter hopes to achieve

11. A standardized test was used to assess the level of depression in a group of patients on a cardiac care unit. The results yielded a mean of 14.60 with confidence interval of 14.55 and 14.65. This presented confidence interval is

A. less precise, but has a higher confidence than 14.20 and 15.00
B. more precise, but has a lower confidence than 14.20 and 15.00
C. less precise, but has a lower confidence than 14.20 and 15.00
D. more precise, but has a higher confidence than 14.20 and 15.00
E. indeterminate, because the degree of confidence is not specified

12. A recently published report explored the relationship between height and subjects' self-reported cholesterol levels in a sample of 44- to 65-year-old males. The report included a correlation of +0.02, computed for the relationship between height and cholesterol level. One of the possible interpretations of this correlation is:

A. The statistic proves that there is no definable relationship between the two specified variables.
B. There is a limited causal relationship between the two specified variables.
C. A real-life relationship may exist, but the measurement error is too large.
D. A scatterplot of the data will show a clear linear slope.
E. The correlation is significant at the 0.02 level.

Question 13–15

The Collaborative Depression study examined several factors impacting the detection and treatment of depression. One primary focus was to develop a biochemical test for diagnosing depression. For this research, a subpopulation of 300 persons was selected and subjected to the dexamethasone suppression test (DST). The results of the study are as follows:

	Actual Depression	
	NO	YES
DST Results		
Depressed	87	102
Nondepressed	63	48

13. Which of these ratios measures specificity?

A. 102:150
B. 102:189
C. 63:150
D. 87:150
E. 63:111

14. Which of these ratios measures positive predictive value?

    A. 102:150
    B. 102:189
    C. 63:150
    D. 87:150
    E. 63:111

15. Which of these ratios measures sensitivity?

    A. 102:150
    B. 102:189
    C. 63:150
    D. 87:150
    E. 63:111

16. Initial research supported a conclusion that a positive relationship exists between coffee consumption and heart disease. However, subsequent, more extensive research suggests that the initial conclusion was the result of a type I error. In this context, a type I error

    A. means there is no real-life significance, but statistical significance is found
    B. suggests that the researcher has probably selected the wrong statistical test
    C. results from a nonexclusionary clause in the null hypothesis
    D. indicates that the study failed to detect an effect statistically, when one is present in the population
    E. has a probability in direct proportion to the size of the test statistic

17. A survey of a popular seaside community (population 1,225) found the local inhabitants to have unusually elevated blood pressure. In this survey, just over 95% of the population had systolics between 110 and 190. Assuming a normal distribution for these assessed blood pressures, the standard deviation for systolic blood pressure in this seaside community is most likely

    A. 10
    B. 20
    C. 30
    D. 40
    E. 50

18. A report of a clinical trial of a new drug for herpes simplex II versus a placebo noted that the new drug gave a higher proportion of success than the placebo. The report ended with the statement: *chi*-square = 4.72, $p < 0.05$. In light of this information, we may conclude that

A. fewer than one in 20 will fail to benefit from the drug

B. the chance that an individual patient will fail to benefit is less than 0.05

C. if the drug were effective, the probability of the reported finding is less than one in 20

D. if the drug were ineffective, the probability of the reported finding is less than 0.05

E. the null hypothesis is false

19. A recent study was conducted to assess the intelligence of students enrolled in an alternative high school program. The results showed the IQs of the students distributed according to the normal curve, with a mean of 115 and a standard deviation of 10. Based on this information it is most reasonable to conclude that

A. 50% of the students will have an IQ below the standard mean of 100

B. 5% of the students will have IQs below 105

C. students with IQs of 125 are at the 84th percentile

D. 2.5% of the students will have IQs greater than 125

E. all of the students' scores fall between 85 and 135

20. A correlation of +0.56 is found between alcohol consumption and systolic blood pressure in men. This correlation is significant at the 0.001 level. From this information we may conclude that:

A. There is no association between alcohol consumption and systolic pressure.

B. Men who consume less alcohol are at lower risk for increased systolic pressure.

C. Men who consume less alcohol are at higher risk for increased systolic pressure.

D. High alcohol consumption can cause increased systolic pressure in men.

E. High systolic pressure can cause increased alcohol consumption in men.

Questions 21-23

To assess the effects of air pollution on health, a random sample of 250 residents of Denver, Colorado, were given thorough checkups every 2 years. This same procedure was followed on a matched sample of persons living in Fort Collins, Colorado, a smaller town located about 60 miles north. Some of the results, presented as percent mortality, are displayed in the table below.

Cumulative Mortality in 2 Communities Over 10 Years

	1975	1977	1979	1981	1983	1985
Denver	4%	6%	10%	15%	22%	28%
Fort Collins	2%	3%	7%	10%	12%	14%

21. This type of study can be best characterized as a

    A. cross-sectional study
    B. clinical case trial design
    C. cross-over study
    D. cohort study
    E. case-control study

22. According to the data presented in the table, the cumulative relative risk for living in Denver by the year 1981 was

    A. 0.67
    B. 5%
    C. 1.5
    D. 2.0
    E. 1.33

23. What statistical test would you run to test whether there was a difference between the cumulative mortality rate for Denver and Fort Collins in 1985?

    A. *t*-test
    B. ANOVA
    C. Regression
    D. Correlation coefficient
    E. *Chi*-square

24. A study is conducted to examine the relationship between myocardial infarction and time spent driving when commuting to and from work. One hundred married males who had suffered infarcts were selected and their average commuting time ascertained from either the subject, or if the infarct had been fatal, their spouse. A comparison group of 100 married males who had not suffered infarcts was also selected and their average commuting time recorded. When examining this data for a possibly causal relationship between commuting time and the occurrence of myocardial infarcts, the most likely measure of association is

   A. odds ratio
   B. relative risk
   C. incidence rate
   D. attributable risk
   E. correlation coefficient

25. A particular association determines membership based on members' IQ scores. Only those people who have documented IQ scores at least 2 standard deviations above the mean on the Wechsler Adult Intelligence Scale, Revised (WAIS-R), are eligible for admission. Out of a group of 400 people randomly selected from the population at large, how many would be eligible for membership in this society?

   A. 2
   B. 4
   C. 6
   D. 8
   E. 10

26. A physician wishes to study whether moderate alcohol consumption is associated with heart disease. If, in reality, moderate alcohol consumption leads to a relative risk of heart disease of 0.60, the physician wants to have a 95% chance of detecting an effect this large in the planned study. This statement is an illustration of specifying

   A. alpha error
   B. beta error
   C. a null hypothesis
   D. criterion odds
   E. statistical power

27. Public health officials were examining a suspicious outbreak of diarrhea in an inner city community child-care center. Center workers identified children with diarrhea and all children at the center were studied. Officials discovered that children who drank liquids from a bottle were more likely to have diarrhea than children who drank from a glass. They concluded that drinking from unclean bottles was the cause of the outbreak. The use of bottles was subsequently banned from the center. The outbreak subsided. Which of the following is the most likely source of bias in this study?

    A. Recall bias
    B. Lead-time bias
    C. Measurement bias
    D. Confounding
    E. Random differences as to the identification of diarrhea

28. Suicides in teenagers in a small Wisconsin town had been a rare event before 11 cases were recorded in 1994. This unusual occurrence led to the initiation of an investigation to try to determine the reason for this upsurge. The researchers suspect that the suicides are linked to the increasing numbers of new families who have recently moved to the town. The best type of study to explore this possibility would likely be a

    A. cohort study
    B. case-control study
    C. cross-over study
    D. cross-sectional study
    E. community trial study

<u>**Questions 29–38**</u>

Which statistical test will most likely be used to analyze the data?

29. Comparing the blood sugar levels of husbands and wives

    A. *t*-test
    B. *Chi*-square test
    C. One-way ANOVA
    D. Two-way ANOVA
    E. Pearson correlation
    F. Matched pairs *t*-test

30. Comparing the number of staff who do or do not call in sick for each of 3 different nursing shifts

    A. *t*-test
    B. *Chi*-square test
    C. One-way ANOVA
    D. Two-way ANOVA
    E. Pearson correlation
    F. Matched pairs *t*-test

31. Relationship between time spent on studying and test score

    A. *t*-test
    B. *Chi*-square test
    C. One-way ANOVA
    D. Two-way ANOVA
    E. Pearson correlation
    F. Matched pairs *t*-test

32. A researcher believes that boys with same-sex siblings are more likely to have higher testosterone levels.

    A. *t*-test
    B. *Chi*-square test
    C. One-way ANOVA
    D. Two-way ANOVA
    E. Pearson correlation
    F. Matched pairs *t*-test

33. A physician believes that drawing blood is faster with a vacutainer for someone once that person is trained, but faster with a standard syringe for someone with no training.

    A. *t*-test
    B. *Chi*-square test
    C. One-way ANOVA
    D. Two-way ANOVA
    E. Pearson correlation
    F. Matched pairs *t*-test

34. Twenty rats are coated with margarine and 20 with butter as part of a study to explore the carcinogenic effects of oleo.

    A. *t*-test
    B. *Chi*-square test
    C. One-way ANOVA
    D. Two-way ANOVA
    E. Pearson correlation
    F. Matched pairs *t*-test

35. To assess the efficacy of surgical interventions for breast cancer, the quality of life, measured on a 10-point scale, of 30 women who underwent radical mastectomies was compared with 30 women who received radiation treatments and 15 women who refused any medical intervention.

A. *t*-test
B. *Chi*-square test
C. One-way ANOVA
D. Two-way ANOVA
E. Pearson correlation
F. Matched pairs *t*-test

36. Comparison of passing and failure rates at each of 3 test sites.

A. *t*-test
B. *Chi*-square test
C. One-way ANOVA
D. Two-way ANOVA
E. Pearson correlation
F. Matched pairs *t*-test

37. Comparison of actual measured test scores for students at each of 3 test sites.

A. *t*-test
B. *Chi*-square test
C. One-way ANOVA
D. Two-way ANOVA
E. Pearson correlation
F. Matched pairs *t*-test

38. Assessing changes in blood pressure for a group of 30 hypertensives 1 week before and 3 months after beginning a course of antihypertensive medication.

A. *t*-test
B. *Chi*-square test
C. One-way ANOVA
D. Two-way ANOVA
E. Pearson correlation
F. Matched pairs *t*-test

39. In a study of chemical workers, 400 workers with respiratory disease and 150 workers without respiratory disease were selected for examination. The investigators obtained a history of exposure to a particular solvent in both groups of workers. Among workers with the respiratory disease, 250 gave a history of exposure to the solvent, compared to 50 of the workers without respiratory disease. The study design can best be described as a

    A. case-control study
    B. cohort study
    C. cross-sectional study
    D. community trial
    E. comparative clinical trial

40. The air quality is assessed in two Midwestern cities, one in which a government program has instituted reducing the amount of carbon monoxide emissions allowed, and one without the government program. The rates of respiratory problems in both cities are recorded over a 5-year period. Given the design of this study, an appropriate one-tailed null hypothesis would be

    A. air quality is related to respiratory problems in both of the cities under study.
    B. air quality is related to respiratory problems in the city with the government program but not in the other city.
    C. no evidence will be found for differences in air quality between the two cities.
    D. the rate of respiratory problems in the city with the government program will not be any lower than that of the other city.
    E. air quality will be inversely related to the rate of respiratory problems in both cities.

Answers and Explanations

9. **Answer: D.** Relative risk means divide, compute the ratio between the 2 groups. [230/71 = 3.2]

10. **Answer: D.** This is a definition question. Null hypothesis is a statement of chance, the opposite of what the researcher hopes to find.

11. **Answer: B.** A smaller interval is more precise but less confident. Precise means *narrower* interval. 95% confidence yields a smaller interval than 99% confidence.

12. **Answer: C.** One reason for a near-zero correlation is that the error of measurement is so large that it obscures an underlying relationship. It shows no linear relationship and does not mean cause. The number given is the coefficient, not *p*-value.

13. **Answer: C.** True negatives, out of all non diseased. [TN/(TN + FP)] = [63/(87 + 63)].

14. **Answer: B.** True positives, out of all positives. [TP/(TP + FP)] = [102/(102 + 87)].

15. **Answer: A.** True positives, out of all diseased. [TP/(TP + FN)] = [102/(102 + 48)].

16. **Answer: A.** A type I error means the researcher rejected the null hypothesis but should not have. This means that although statistical significance is found, there is no real-world significance. By reversing the clauses in the answer, the correct answer becomes more apparent. Answer choice D is a good definition of a type II error.

17. **Answer: B.** If 95% of cases fall between 110 and 190 and the distribution is symmetrical, then the mean must be 150, and the numbers given are 2 standard deviations above and below the mean. This means that 2 standard deviations must equal 40 and that one standard deviation equals 20.

18. **Answer: D.** The key here is the "p-value." Ignore the *chi*-square value. If less than 0.05, this gives the chance of a type I error. Therefore, the probability of the finding if the drug was ineffective.

19. **Answer: C.** This is one standard deviation above the mean. [115 + 10]. Below this point are 84% of the cases using the normal curve.

20. **Answer: B.** The given correlation is statistically significant at the 0.001 level and can therefore be interpreted. It is a positive correlation, suggesting that high goes with high and low goes with low. Avoid answers which suggest a causal relationship.

21. **Answer: D.** People in the 2 communities are followed forward in time, and incidence (mortality) is the outcome.

22. **Answer: C.** The key is to focus only on 1981. Relative risk means divide. [15%/10% = 1.5] or 1.5 times the risk.

23. **Answer: E.** Denver versus Fort Collins is one nominal variable with 2 groups. Dead versus alive is the second nominal variable. Two nominal variables with $n > 25$ = *chi*-square.

24. **Answer: A.** This is a case-control study (infarcts versus no infarcts). Therefore, use an odds ratio. The data is not incidence data, so relative risk does not apply.

25. **Answer: E.** The IQ is scaled to have a mean of 100 and a standard deviation of 15. What percent of the cases are more than 2 standard deviations above the mean? (2.5%) Therefore, what is 2.5% of 400? (10)

26. **Answer: E.** Power is the chance of detecting a difference in the study if there really is a difference in the real world. The question tells us what chance the researcher will have of finding a difference.

27. **Answer: D.** Bottle versus glass is confounded with age or maturity. The other options, while possible, are unlikely.

28. **Answer: B.** Select suicide cases and compare with nonsuicides (controls).

29. **Answer: F.** Blood sugar levels are ratio data, treated as interval data. Husbands and wives are nominal, but are linked nonindependent, matched pairs; therefore, matched pairs *t*-test.

30. **Answer: B.** Staff either call in sick or do not (nominal variable) over 3 shifts (nominal variable). Two nominal variables with a 2 × 3 design, *chi*-square.

31. **Answer: E.**"Is there a relationship?" between 2 interval level variables. Pearson correlation.

32. **Answer: A.** Same sex versus no same sex (nominal variable). Testosterone level is assessed as ratio and treated as interval. Therefore, simple *t*-test.

33. **Answer: D.** Vacutainer versus standard syringe (nominal), training versus no training (nominal), and time (interval). Two nominal and one interval = two-way ANOVA.

34. **Answer: B.** Margarine versus butter (nominal), cancer versus no cancer (nominal). Therefore, *chi*-square.

35. **Answer: C.** There are 3 types of treatment: surgery, radiation, and none (nominal variable, 3 groups), quality of life on the given scale (interval). Therefore, one-way ANOVA.

36. **Answer: B.** Passing versus failure (nominal), 3 sites (nominal). Therefore, *chi*-square.

37. **Answer: C.** Three sites (nominal) with actual test scores (interval). Therefore, one-way ANOVA.

38. **Answer: F.** Before and after (nominal, two-groups, matched pairs), and blood pressure (interval). Therefore, matched pairs *t*-test.

39. **Answer: A.** Respiratory (cases) versus nonrespiratory disease (controls), looking at history.

40. **Answer: D.** The correct statement needs to be a one-directional statement of no effect. "Not any lower than" satisfies this criterion.

SECTION II

Behavioral Science

Substance-Related Disorders 3

Learning Objectives

- ❏ Use knowledge of physiology of substance-related disorders
- ❏ Use knowledge of alcohol and alcoholism
- ❏ Demonstrate understanding of common abused substances
- ❏ Explain information related to other abused substances
- ❏ Demonstrate understanding of substance-abusing physicians

PHYSIOLOGY OF SUBSTANCE-RELATED DISORDERS

The addiction pathway in the brain is a dopamine pathway. Activation of this pathway accounts for the "positive reinforcement" feeling and makes one want to repeat the action which triggered that feeling.

Mesolimbic pathway

Stimulus → Cerebral Cortex → Ventral Tegmental Area → Nucleus Accumbens

- food
- drugs
- sex
- kindness

Dopamine (↑ desire for stimulus)

Serotonin (gives body the impression of satisfaction so cravings are reduced)

Drugs that work in the **nucleus accumbens** include amphetamines, cocaine, opiates, **THC**, PCP, nicotine, and ketamine. Drugs that work in the **ventral tegmental** area include opiates, alcohol, barbiturates, and benzodiazepines.

ALCOHOL

Alcoholism is the most expensive health problem in the United States, costing over $100 billion a year for alcohol-related illness and death. Since 1980, the per capita consumption of alcohol has declined. Nevertheless, tobacco accounts for more loss of life. The best way to reduce long-term mortality is to eliminate smoking.

- Alcohol is most abused drug for all ages; ~10% of all adults are problem drinkers (M > W)
- Alcohol is most widely used illicit drug for teenagers (marijuana is most widely used illicit drug overall)
- Binge drinking is becoming more common; proportion of heavy drinkers age <20 has increased
- Alcoholism rates are higher for low-SES groups though they recover sooner

Note

Crime is the major cost issue for illegal drugs.

Alcohol use has been implicated in 15% of all car accidents, and in 50% of all car accidents not involving a pedestrian, auto accident deaths, homicides (killer or victim), and hospital admissions.

There is increasing evidence for a genetic contribution in alcoholism. Concordance rates are MZ > DZ (MZ 60%, DZ 30%), with marked ethnic-group differences as follows:

- Asian-, Jewish-, and Italian-Americans are much less likely to develop alcoholism than Americans with northern European roots.
- Capacity to tolerate alcohol is the key (enzyme induction, lack of tyrosine kinase).
- If biologic father was an alcoholic, the incidence of alcoholism in males adopted into nonalcoholic families is equal to the incidence of alcoholism in sons raised by biologic alcoholic fathers.
- Family history of alcoholism increases likelihood of major depression in offspring.

The **CAGE** questionnaire is a widely used screening test for problem drinking and potential alcoholism.

- Have you ever tried to **C**ut down on alcohol intake and not succeeded?
- Have you ever been **A**nnoyed about criticism concerning your drinking?
- Have you ever felt **G**uilty about your drinking behavior?
- Have you ever had to take a drink as an **E**ye-opener in the morning to relieve the anxiety and shakiness?

Medical complications of alcohol abuse include cirrhosis, alcoholic hepatitis, pancreatitis, gastric or duodenal ulcer, esophageal varices, middle-age onset of diabetes, GI cancer, hypertension, peripheral neuropathies, myopathies, cardiomyopathy, cerebral vascular accident, erectile dysfunction, vitamin deficiencies, pernicious anemia, and brain disorders, including Wernicke-Korsakoff syndrome (mortality rate of untreated Wernicke is 50%; treatment is with thiamine). Chronic alcohol use can lead to cognitive decline.

Fetal alcohol syndrome (FAS), a group of conditions that may result from a mother's alcohol consumption while pregnant, is the **leading known cause of intellectual disability** (Down syndrome is second). Consumption of large quantities of alcohol is needed to produce FAS; it is characterized by developmental and intellectual disability, craniofacial abnormalities, and limb dislocation.

The most successful way to get an alcoholic into **treatment** is referral by an employer. Alcoholics Anonymous, the original 12-step program and the largest source of alcohol treatment in the United States, is a spiritual program with regular meetings and sponsors who provide substitute dependency, social support, and external reminders that drinking is aversive. Al-Anon, for family and friends, deals with codependence and enabling behaviors.

The stages of behaviorial change related to alcoholism are :

- **Precontemplation**: unaware of problem
- **Contemplation**: aware of problem but ambivalent about action
- **Preparation**: first decision to change; small steps taken
- **Action**: change begins; trial and error
- **Maintenance**: new behaviors practiced; focus on relapse prevention
- **Relapse**: efforts to change abandoned

The cycle may repeat until sobriety is established.

Pharmacologic treatments include naltrexone (reduces cravings) and disulfiram (reduces alcohol consumption), which works by inhibiting aldehyde dehydrogenase. However, it produces symptoms of nausea, chest pain, hyperventilation, tachycardia, and vomiting. and should be used with psychotherapy (or 12-step program). It is based on aversive conditioning.

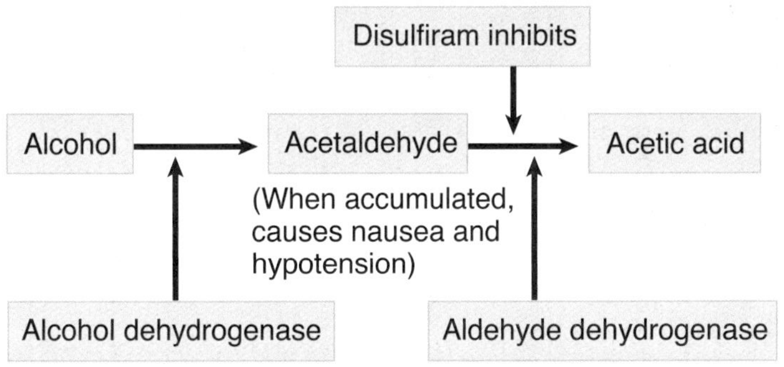

Figure 3-1. Disulfiram Treatment

COMMON ABUSED SUBSTANCES

Table 3-1. Summary of Substance Abuse

Substance	Intoxication	Withdrawal	Treatment	Psychopharmacology
Amphetamines (release DA) Cocaine (prevent re-uptake of DA)	Euphoria, hypervigilance, anxiety, stereotyped behavior, grandiosity, paranoia, tachycardia, pupillary dilation	Depression, fatigue, increased appetite unpleasant dreams, suicide	Antipsychotics or benzodi-azepines for intoxication; bromocriptine, amantadine, bupropion for withdrawal	Noradrenaline system, NAC pathway (dopaminergic)
Caffeine	Restlessness, agitation, insomnia, diuresis, GI disturbances, excitement	Headache, fatigue, drowsiness, nausea or vomiting (1–4 days)	Analgesics for withdrawal	Antagonist of adenosine recep-tors, increased cAMP in neurons that have adenosine receptors
Cannabis (e.g., marijuana, hashish)	Impaired motor coordination, anxiety, slowed reaction time, impaired judg-ment, conjunctival injection, dry mouth, increased appetite, psychosis	None	Abstinence and support	Inhibitory G protein, GABA, increased serotonin, lower level of NAC activation
Hallucinogens (e.g., LSD, mescaline, ketamine)	Hallucinations, illusions, anxiety, ideas of reference, depersonalization, pupillary dilation, tremors, uncoordination	None	Supportive counseling, talking down, antipsychotics or benzo-diazepines for intoxication	Partial agonist at postsynaptic 5-HT receptors
Inhalants (glue, paint thinner)	Belligerence, impaired judgment, nystag-mus, uncoordination, lethargy, unsteady gait, crusting around nose/mouth	None	Education and counseling	GABA, cross tolerance, cerebellum (versus basal ganglia for Parkinson's)
Nicotine	None in usual doses but more depression (2×), impotency, traffic accidents, and more days lost from work	Irritability, depressed mood and heart rate, increased appetite, insomnia, anxiety	Nicotine patch, education, bupropion, varenicline, bromocriptine	Agonist at Ach receptors, activates dopaminergic pathway (positive reinforcer),speeds and intensifies flow of glutamate
Opiates (heroin, codeine, oxycodone)	Pupillary constriction, constipation, drowsiness, slurred speech, respiratory depression, bradycardia, coma, death	"Flu-like" muscle aches, nausea or vomiting, yawning, piloerection, lacrimation, rhinorrhea, fever, insomnia, pupillary dilation (7–10 days)	For intoxication naloxone (short half-life); clonidine, methadone, buprenorphine for withdrawal	Opiate receptors, locus cereleus pathway (noradrenergic), NAC pathway
Phencyclidine (PCP, angel dust)	Assaultive, combative, impulsive, agitated, nystagmus, ataxia, hypersaliva-tion, muscle rigidity, decreased response to pain, hyperacusis, paranoia, unpredictible violence, psychosis	None	Nonstimulating environment, restraints, vitamin C, benzodiazepines, or antipsychotics for intoxication	Antagonist of N-methyl D-aspartate glutamate receptors, prevents influx of calcium ions, activates dopaminergic neurons
Sedative hypnotics (barbituates, benzodiazepines)	Impaired judgment, slurred speech, unco-ordination, unsteady gait, stupor, coma, death–barb confusion, falls, memory problems for benzos	Autonomic hyperactivity tremors, hyperactivity; hallucinations, anxiety, grand mal seizures, death	Mechanical ventilation in overdose; sodium bicarbonate to alkanize urine in barbituate overdose	GABA, cross-tolerance, delirium

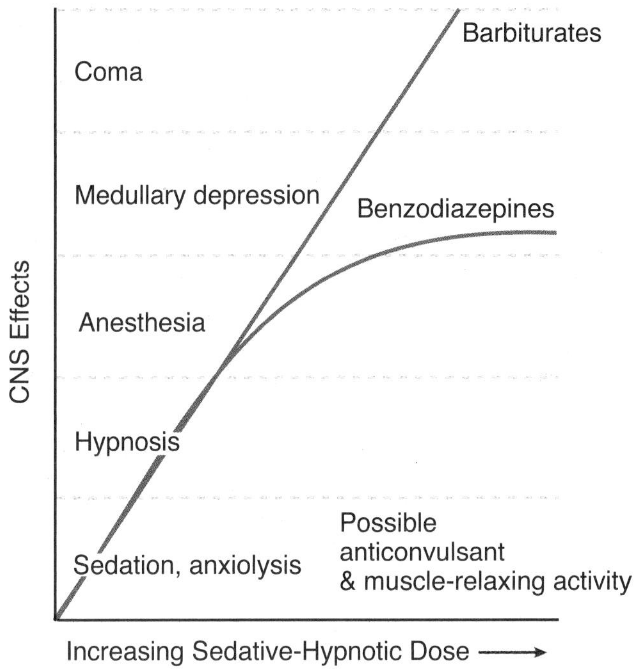

OTHER ABUSED SUBSTANCES

Most illicit drug users are employed full-time. Men > women roughly 2.5 to 1.

About 33% of psychiatric disorders are substance-related. The prevalence of substance-related disorders in newly admitted psychiatric inpatients or outpatients is roughly 50%; these "dual diagnosis" patients are very difficult to treat and tend to continue use when on inpatient wards. Substance-related disorders adds to the suicide risk of any underlying psychiatric diagnosis.

About 50% of emergency department visits are substance-related. Physicians tend to underdiagnose substance-related problems of all types, especially those in women, high-SES patients, and other physicians.

Ecstasy (MDMA)

Also called "E," X, or XTC, ecstasy acts as a hallucinogen combined with an amphetamine. Effects begin in 45 minutes and last 2–4 hours. Symptoms include derealization, hallucinations, mania-like mood, hyperthermia, hypertension, fatigue the day after use, convulsions, and possible death.

Anabolic Steroids

Anabolic steroids are taken by athletes to increase performance and physique. With chronic use they can cause cardiomyopathy, bone mineral loss with later osteoporosis, hypertension, diabetes, atrophy of testis, mood lability, depression, and atypical psychosis. Presenting signs include skin atrophy, spontaneous bruising, acne, low serum potassium levels.

- **Men** may experience breast development, scrotal pain, or premature baldness.
- **Women** may experience disrupted menstrual cycle, deepening of voice, or excessive body hair.

Table 3-2. Helpful Hints of Substance-Related Disorders

Paranoia	Cocaine/amphetamine intoxication
Depression	Cocaine/amphetamine withdrawal
Arrhythmias	Cocaine intoxication
Violence	PCP
Vertical nystagmus	PCP
Pinpoint pupils	Opiate overdose (treatment = naloxone)
Flu-like	Opiate withdrawal (treatment = clonidine)
Flashbacks	LSD
Seizures	Benzodiazepine/alcohol withdrawal
Death	Barbiturate withdrawal

SUBSTANCE ABUSE BY PHYSICIANS

Physician impairment issues are dealt with by the state licensing boards. Psychiatrists and anesthesiologists have the highest rates of substance abuse.

If you suspect that a colleague has a substance-related problem, do the following **in this order**:

1. Get the colleague to suspend patient contact.
2. Report it to hospital administration and the state board.
3. Ideally, get the colleague into treatment.

Review Questions

1. The medical record of a 65-year-old white man details a long list of medical conditions, including diabetes, gastric ulcer, recurrent headache, and peripheral neuropathies. A history of substance-related disorder is also documented, though no specifics are provided. When interviewing the patient, the physician is most likely to discover that the substance abused by the patient most likely was

   A. alcohol
   B. cocaine
   C. caffeine
   D. ecstasy
   E. hallucinogens
   F. inhalants
   G. opiates
   H. sedative hypnotics

2. A 21-year-old man is brought to the emergency department by his parents, who are concerned because he was stumbling around their house, waving his arms, and verbally unresponsive to their questions. Upon examination the patient appears anxious, with elevated heart rate and clammy skin. A slight tremor is evident in the hands and the pupils are dilated. Over time, the patient becomes verbal and reports feeling like he was floating "out of body," and that words spoken to him seemed like insects that should be swatted away. He also admits to having recently taken an illegal substance. The patient's behavior and physiology are most consistent with intoxication due to

   A. cocaine
   B. inhaled paint thinner
   C. marijuana
   D. mescaline
   E. phencyclidine
   F. phenobarbital

3. The police bring a 22-year-old white man to the emergency department. From the outset, he is belligerent, aggressive, and violent, requiring the efforts of several officers to restrain him. When questioned, the patient is paranoid. Physical exam shows him to have muscle rigidity and pupils that move up and down rapidly. The patient had previously been treated for opiate overdose. What neurochemical mechanisms are most likely to account for the patient's current behavior?

   A. Reduction in levels of GABA
   B. Antagonism of the glutamate receptors
   C. Partial agonist of the postsynaptic serotonin receptors
   D. Antagonism of the locus cerelose pathway and blocking of substance P
   E. Increases in GABA and inhibitory G protein

4. Parents bring their 17-year-old son to the emergency department because he is "just not himself." Preliminary examination shows the boy to be drowsy, with slurred speech, pupillary constriction, lethargy, and generally positive affect. The boy is most likely intoxicated with which of the following?

   A. Caffeine
   B. Cannabis
   C. Cocaine
   D. LSD
   E. Alcohol
   F. Inhalants
   G. Phencyclidine
   H. Nicotine
   I. Opiates
   J. Sedative hypnotics

Answers and Explanations

1. **Answer: A.** Alcohol is the most abused drug for any age. Note that the patient's symptoms, with the exception of the headache, are all linked to long-term alcohol use.

2. **Answer: D.** The patient presents behavior and symptoms of someone high on hallucinogens. Although cocaine may also induce anxiety, the case lacks the other cocaine-related symptoms.

3. **Answer: B.** The presenting profile is most suggestive of PCP intoxication, which produces its behavioral effects by antagonism of the glutamate receptors and the activation of dopamine neurons.

4. **Answer: I.** Pupillary constriction and lethargy are the key features here.

Human Sexuality 4

Learning Objectives

- ❑ Use knowledge of sexual behavior in the United States
- ❑ Demonstrate understanding of paraphilic disorders, sexual dysfunction, masturbation, and homosexuality
- ❑ Explain how sexuality and aging are related

SEXUAL BEHAVIOR IN THE UNITED STATES

In the United States, 95% of people have their first sexual experience outside of marriage.

Adolescent Sexual Behavior

By age 19 nearly 70% of all unmarried women and 80% of men are nonvirgins. The average age of first sexual experience is 16. Adolescents in the aggregate drift into sexual activity rather than decide to have sex. Most adolescent sexual activity takes place in the context of one primary relationship; most adolescents are not promiscuous, but "serially monogamous."

Nearly 4 in 10 teenage girls whose first intercourse experience happened at age 13–14 report that the sex was unwanted or involuntary.

According to a recent survey, 57% of adolescents claim to have used a condom the last time they had sex, though other research suggests they do not do as they say. More than 50% of sexually active adolescents do not use birth control regularly.

Teenage Pregnancy

Teenagers today are less sexually active than they used to be, but those who are will most likely use birth control.

- 10% of teenagers become pregnant each year
- About 80% of these pregnancies are unintended and outside of marriage
- Teenage pregnancy among girls age <15 has been increasing.

In 2014 approximately 249,000 babies were born in the United States to women age 15–19. This reflects a decrease for teens in this age group.

- 50% of all unwed mothers are teenagers.
- 50% have the child, 33% have elective abortion, and the remainder are spontaneously aborted
- About 33% of girls aged 15–19 have at least 1 unwanted pregnancy.
- Single mothers account for 70% of births to girls aged 15–19.

For the **mother**, the consequences of teenage pregnancy include a high risk for obstetric complications (leading cause of school dropout). For the **child**, consequences include possible lower level of intellectual functioning and problems of the single-parent family (increased risk of delinquency, suicide). Neonatal deaths and prematurity are common.

Sexually Transmitted Diseases

One in 5 teenagers will have a sexually transmitted disease (STD); rates for gonorrhea and chlamydia are higher for adolescents than for any older group.

- Highest incidence: most common STD is **human papilloma virus (HPV)**
- Highest prevalence: one in 5 Americans has herpes simplex virus, type 2 (HSV-2)
- In women, chlamydia is the most commonly reported STD; in men, gonorrhea
- Syphilis (primary and secondary) cases have doubled since 1970; rate now more than 20/100,000
- Number of gonorrhea cases has declined by half since 1975; increase in resistant strains since 1975

Normal Sexual Response Cycle

Table 4-1. Male Sexual Response Cycle

Body Area	Excitement Phase	Orgasm Phase	Resolution Phase
Skin	Sexual flush	3–15 seconds	Disappears
Penis	Vasocongestion, penile erection	Ejaculation	Detumescence
Scrotum	Tightening and lifting	No change	Decrease to baseline size
Testes	Elevation and increase in size	No change	Decrease to baseline size, descent
Breasts	Nipple erection	No change	Return to baseline

During the excitement and orgasm phase, there is an increase in respiration, tachycardia up to 180 beats/minute, rise in systolic blood pressure 20–100 mm Hg and diastolic blood pressure 10–50 mm Hg.

Table 4-2. Female Sexual Response Cycle

Body Area	Excitement Phase	Orgasm Phase	Resolution Phase
Skin	Sexual flush	3–15 seconds	Disappears
Breasts	Nipple erection, areolas enlarge	May become tremulous	Return to normal
Clitoris	Enlargement, shaft retracts	No change	Detumescence, shaft returns to normal
Labia majora	Nulliparous: elevate and flatten Multiparous: congestion and edema	No change	Nulliparous: increase to normal size Multiparous: decrease to normal size
Labia minora	Increase in size, deeper in color	Contractions of proximal portion	Return to normal
Vagina	Transudate, elongation	Contractions in lower third 1/3	Congestion disappears, ejaculate forms seminal pool in upper 2/3
Uterus	Ascends into false pelvis "Tenting effect"	Contractions	Contractions cease and uterus descends

PARAPHILIC DISORDERS

Pedophilia: sexual urges toward children; most common paraphilia

Exhibitionism: recurrent desire to expose genitals to stranger

Voyeurism: sexual pleasure from watching others who are naked, grooming, or having sex; begins early in childhood

Sadism: sexual pleasure derived from others' pain

Masochism: sexual pleasure derived from being abused or dominated

Fetishism: sexual focus on objects, e.g., shoes, stockings; transvestite fetishism involves fantasies or actual dressing by heterosexual men in female clothes for sexual arousal

Frotteurism: male rubbing of genitals against fully clothed woman to achieve orgasm; subways and buses

Zoophilia: animals preferred in sexual fantasies or practices

Coprophilia: combining sex and defecation

Urophilia: combining sex and urination

Necrophilia: preferred sex with cadavers

Hypoxyphilia: altered state of consciousness secondary to hypoxia while experiencing orgasm; achieved with autoerotic asphyxiation, poppers, amyl nitrate, nitric oxide

Table 4-3. Gender Identity and Preferred Sexual Partner of a Biologic Male

Common Label	Gender Identity	Preferred Sexual Partner
Heterosexual	Male	Female
Transvestite fetishism	Male	Female
Gender dysphoria (transsexual)	Female	Male
Homosexual	Male	Male

Gender identity: sense of maleness or femaleness, established by age 3.

SEXUAL DYSFUNCTION

Sexual Desire Disorders

In **male hypoactive sexual desire disorder**, men experience a deficiency or absence of fantasies or desires. Reasons: low testosterone, CNS depressants, common postsurgery, depression, marital discord.

Sexual Arousal Disorders

In **female sexual interest/arousal disorder,** women are unable to achieve adequate vaginal lubrication. Reasons: possible hormonal connection (many women report peak sexual desire just prior to menses), antihistamine and anticholinergic medications which can reduce vaginal lubrication

Male erectile disorder (impotence) has 10–20% lifetime prevalence; point prevalence is 3%. Half of men treated for sexual disorder complain of impotence. Incidence is 8% young adult and 75% men age >80. The disorder is 50% more likely in smokers. Be sure to check alcohol usage, diabetes, marital conflict, as it must be determined whether the cause is organic or psychological.

Assessment: postage stamp test, snap gauge (to test physiological versus psychological).

Treatment is sildenafil (Viagra), vardenafil (Levitra), tadalafil (Cialis).

Orgasm Disorders

Female orgasm disorder is an inability to achieve orgasm. 5% of married women age >35 have never achieved orgasm. Overall prevalence from all causes is 30%. Treatment is fantasy, vibrators.

In **premature ejaculation**, the male ejaculates before or immediately after entering vagina. It is more common if early sexual experiences were in back seat of car or were with prostitute, or there is anxiety about sexual act. Treatment is stop-and-go technique, squeeze technique, SSRIs.

Genitopelvic Pain/Penetration Disorders

Genitopelvic pain/penetration disorders involve involuntary muscle constriction of the outer third of the vagina which prevents penile insertion. Psychological in origin, they involve recurrent and persistent pain before, during, or after intercourse. These disorders are only diagnosed in women, and not diagnosed if caused by medical conditions. Treatment is relaxation, Hegar dilator.

MASTURBATION

Masturbation is a normal activity from infancy to old age. The reasons for adults are loneliness, tiredness, boredom, stress relief, and sleep aid. The reasons for children are normal development and it feels good.

- Frequency: 3–4x weekly for adolescents, 1–2x weekly for adults, 1x month for married people
- Men = women
- Abnormal only if interferes with sexual or occupational functioning
- Can lead to premature ejaculation in males who use it primarily to reduce tension

HOMOSEXUALITY

Homosexuality is not considered a mental illness; 4–10% of all males and 1–3% of all females are homosexual. The main issue is partner preference, not behavior. Behavioral patterns of homosexuals are as varied as those of heterosexuals.

- Male–male relationships are less stable than are female–female relationships
- Over 50% of homosexuals have children
- **Ego-syntonic homosexuality** agrees with one's sense of self (person is comfortable), while **ego-dystonic homosexuality** disagrees with sense of self, (makes person uncomfortable/distressed).
- NOT considered pathologic unless ego-dystonic

There is increasing evidence of biologic contribution; higher concordance rates for MZ twins (52%) than for DZ (22%). Preference is well established by adolescence.

- Feelings of preference emerge 3 or more years before first encounter
- Describe duration of feelings with "As long as I can remember"
- Similar number of heterosexual experiences reported in childhood and adolescence; report experiences as "ungratifying"
- 30–40% of all people report at least 1 same-gender sexual experience

SEXUALITY AND AGING

Sexual interest does not decline significantly with aging. Continued sexual interest means sexual activity can continue. The best predictor of sexual activity in the elderly is availability of a partner.

After myocardial infarction (MI), the sexual position that puts least strain on the heart is partner on top.

Changes in men:

- Slower erection
- Longer refractory period
- More stimulation needed

Changes in women:

- Vaginal dryness
- Vaginal thinning
- Can be reduced by estrogen replacement

REVIEW QUESTIONS

1. A young couple visits their physician for counseling soon after they are married. They say they have read that marital satisfaction changes over the course of the marriage and want to know what they should expect as their marriage progresses. The physician tells them that, while their personal experience may be different, overall marital satisfaction tends to

   A. increase with length of time married
   B. decrease with length of time married
   C. increase gradually, reaching a high point when children are in adolescence, then decline rapidly
   D. decrease gradually during the childbearing years, then increases after all children have left home
   E. increase during the preschool years, decreasing during grammar school, then rise again during adolescence

2. Your schedule indicates that you have an initial appointment with a patient who is a 50-year-old white man. Following the examination, the most likely resultant diagnosis for this man is

   A. gastrointestinal problems
   B. upper respiratory distress
   C. essential hypertension
   D. obesity
   E. urinary problems

3. According to surveys by the Centers for Disease Control and Prevention, as of 2000, the most common health problem in the United States is

   A. cancer
   B. heart disease
   C. substance-related disorder
   D. obesity
   E. dental caries

4. A 32-year-old white woman appears at your office for her annual physical exam. The physical exam shows the patient to be in good health, although she is slightly overweight and has moderately elevated blood pressure. If the patient were to die at some point in the next 10 years, the most likely cause of death would be

   A. unintended injuries
   B. neoplasms
   C. heart disease
   D. homicide
   E. AIDS

5. During a 1-year period, a physician practicing medicine in the United States would be most likely to encounter a patient suffering from which of the following mandatory reportable diseases?

   A. Hepatitis A
   B. Lyme disease
   C. HIV/AIDS
   D. Chicken pox
   E. Syphilis

6. An earthquake devastates a town in northern California. Electricity is shut off for several days, and many of the people in the area are homeless. The most likely pattern of response of the affected population would be

   A. widespread emotional aftereffects that are usually mild and transitory
   B. disintegration of social organization
   C. incidence of post-traumatic stress syndrome in close to 20% of those affected
   D. children adapt to the new circumstances more quickly than do adults
   E. increased divorce in the following 6 months

7. You have been appointed to provide an assessment of the general health status of your local community. You have a limited budget and must, therefore, focus on the most likely determinant of community health status. Based on this information, your assessment should focus on

   A. hospital bed:population ratio
   B. infant mortality rate
   C. physician:patient ratio
   D. general mortality rate
   E. quality of the physical and social environment

8. Following surgery for the removal of her appendix, a patient visits her physician complaining of a lack of interest in sexual contact with her husband. "We have been fighting so much lately," she says. "Between that and the pressure I feel at work, I just don't know what to do anymore." Medical history shows that she has been taking diazepam for the past 2 years and oral contraceptives for the past 5 years. Which of the following can be safely excluded as unlikely to result in the reported suppression of libido?

   A. Oral contraceptives
   B. Marital discord
   C. Postoperative recovery
   D. Work stress
   E. Diazepam

9. At the conclusion of her annual gynecologic exam, a 34-year-old married Hispanic woman confides to her physician that her interest in sex has been "spotty" lately. Although she has sexual relations with her husband at least 1x week, she reports feeling "really passionate" only in the week just prior to the onset of menses. She refrains from sexual intercourse during menses. The woman wants to know what is wrong with her. The physician's best response would be

   A. "What medications are you taking?"
   B. "Is your husband sometimes abusive?"
   C. "This is a normal pattern of sexual arousal reported by many women."
   D. "You may find that an erotic movie will stimulate your sexual desire at times when you do not feel passionate."
   E. "How often does your husband want to have sex?"
   F. "I'm going to have you talk to a friend of mine who specializes in this sort of thing."
   G. "You might consider abstaining from sex for awhile until you feel more sure that you want it."

10. A woman reports to her physician that she can achieve orgasm only when recalling a previous, abusive boyfriend. Suspecting the presence of a paraphilia, the physician should explore for further evidence of

   A. coprophilia
   B. transvestitism
   C. sadism
   D. frotteurism
   E. voyeurism
   F. exhibitionism
   G. pedophilia
   H. fetishism
   I. masochism
   J. zoophilia
   K. necrophilia

11. A 72-year-old married man who is being treated for elevated cholesterol asks his physician about normal sexual function in the elderly. At this point, the physician should inform the patient that

   A. loss of interest in sex is a natural part of aging
   B. although men maintain interest in sexual activity, women lose interest as they age
   C. more mental and physical stimulation may be required to achieve erection
   D. sexual activity should be limited to once a month to reduce cardiovascular stress
   E. he will be provided with a prescription for an anti-impotence drug so that it is available when he needs it

Answers and Explanations

1. **Answer: D.** Marital satisfaction tends to be lower for couples with children, and to rise when the children leave home.

2. **Answer: C.** Essential hypertension is the most likely diagnosis resulting from an office visit by a male to his physicians.

3. **Answer: E.** The key here is the phrase "health problem." More people have dental cavities than anything else listed.

4. **Answer: B.** For males in the same age range, the leading cause of death is accidents.

5. **Answer: D.** In order from most to least likely: chicken pox, HIV/AIDS, syphilis, salmonella, hepatitis A.

6. **Answer: A.** The aftermath of natural disasters finds many people suffering from distress reactions. These reactions, however, tend to be relatively mild and resolve themselves of their own accord and generally fall under the diagnosis of acute stress disorder. After natural disasters, there tends to be an increase in social organization. PTSD incidence is closer to 4%. Adults adapt more quickly than children. Divorce rates tend to decline in the period just after a disaster.

7. **Answer: E.** The quality of the overall environment is the main issue. The other, technical sounding, options are all indicators of community health, but are not the most important determinant. Infant mortality is one of the strongest predictors of life expectancy, but not of overall health of the community.

8. **Answer: E.** Although the other items have been shown to suppress sexual desire, diazepam has not.

9. **Answer: C.** Many women report peak sexual arousal just prior to the onset of menses. Reassure the woman that her experience is normal. She needs reassurance, not problem solving or medical intervention.

10. **Answer: I.** To qualify for masochism, the sexual act must be the result of gratification that includes receiving pain in either reality or fantasy.

11. **Answer: C.** Sexual interest does not decline with age for men or women. A prescription should not be given without an identified problem.

Learning and Behavior Modification 5

Learning Objectives

- ❑ Describe the major learning theories and explain how they predict behavior change
- ❑ Explain information related to behavior therapy and behavior modification

LEARNING AND BEHAVIOR

In the behaviorist model of learning and behavior modification, all that matters is the objective data, i.e., only what can be seen, observed, and measured. Internal states, subjective impressions, and unconscious processes are not relevant. The behaviorist definition of learning is a relatively permanent change in behavior, not due to fatigue, drugs, or maturation.

The 2 main types of learning paradigm are **classical (elicited) conditioning** and **operant (emitted) conditioning**.

Classical Conditioning

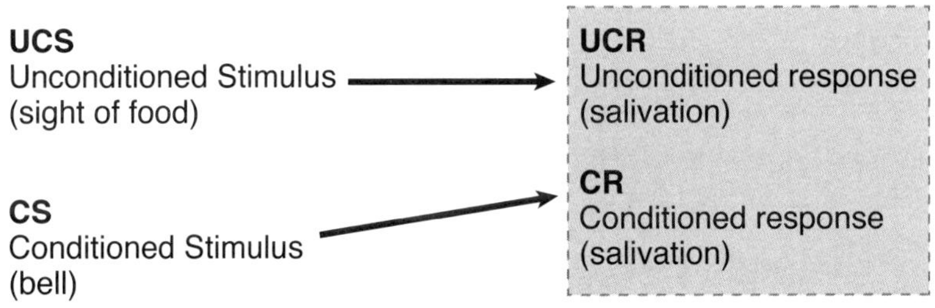

Figure 5-1. Classic (or Respondent or Pavlovian) Conditioning

In **classical conditioning**, the conditioned response is elicited by the conditioned stimulus after repeated pairings of the UCS and CS. The classic example is the Pavlovian experiment, which pairs the ringing of a bell with the bringing of food so that, eventually, the sound of the bell elicits the salivatory response, which previously occurred only with the sight of the food. Or, for example, say a patient receives chemotherapy (UCS), which induces nausea (UCR). Eventually, the sights and sounds of the hospital alone (CS) elicit nausea (now a CR).

- **A new stimulus elicits the same behavior.** Note that the triggering stimulus (CS) occurs before the response.

- **Stimulus generalization:** the tendency for the conditioned stimulus to evoke similar responses after the response has been conditioned. If a salivation response had been conditioned to a tone of 1,000 CPS, an 800 CPS tone will elicit a similar response. Or, in the second example, generalization will have occurred if any hospital, or even meeting a physician, comes to elicit nausea from the patient.
- **Extinction:** after learning has occurred, removal of the pairing between the UCS and the CS results in a decreased probability that the conditioned response will be made. For example, breaking the pairing between chemotherapy and the medical setting by giving chemotherapy at home. The nausea-eliciting properties of hospitals will be extinguished.

Operant or Instrumental Conditioning

In **operant conditioning**, a new response is emitted, perhaps randomly at first, which results in a consequence. The consequence acts as reinforcement and changes the probability of the response's future occurrence. In the Skinner experiment, pressing a lever resulted in the delivery of food. After receiving food, the bar-pressing behavior increased. Because it changed behavior, the food is a reinforcing event.

A new response occurs to an old stimulus. Note the triggering stimulus (reinforcement) occurs after the response.

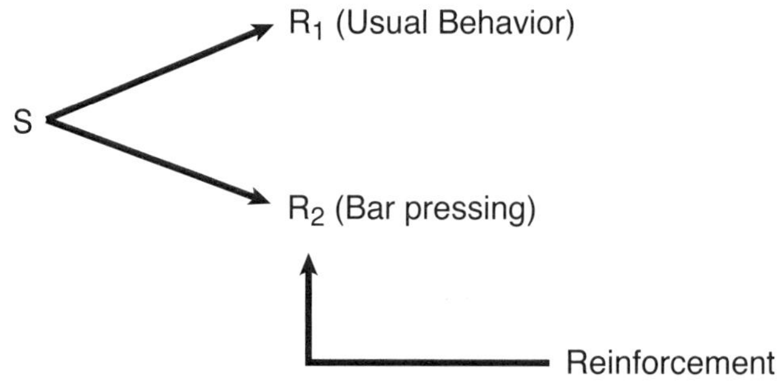

Figure 5-2. Operant or Instrumental Conditioning

Reinforcement is delivery of a consequence that increases the likelihood that a response will occur. A reinforcer is defined by its effects. Any stimulus is a reinforcer if it increases the probability of a response.

A **positive reinforcer** is a stimulus that, when applied following an operant response, strengthens the probability of that response occurring.

- Increased pay leads to increased work from an employee
- Increased complaining leads to increased attention from the nursing staff

A **negative reinforcer** is a stimulus that, when removed following an operant response, strengthens the probability of that response occurring.

- A child learns that he can stop his parents' nagging by cleaning up his room.
- Aversive stimuli such as a loud noise, bright light, shock, can often be negative reinforcers

Positive and negative do not imply good and bad, respectively. Rather, **positive means adding a stimulus** and **negative means removing a stimulus**. Both positive and negative reinforcement lead to an increase in response frequency or strength.

Punishment, like negative conditioning, usually uses a noxious stimulus. However, this stimulus is imposed to weaken response. Ordinarily, punishment should be paired with positive reinforcement for alternative behaviors.

- Physical punishment of a child will suppress naughty behavior, but may fade when the punishment is removed and may model aggressive physical behavior for the child

Extinction refers to the disappearance of a response when it is no longer being reinforced.

- A nurse who is bombarded by constant complaints from a patient stops paying attention to the patient whenever he complains
- A child is ignored by the parents when he throws temper tantrums.
- If successful, the unwanted behavior will stop.

Table 5-1. Types of Reinforcement

		Stimulus: (S)	
		Add	Remove
Behavior: (R)	Stops	Punishment	Extinction
	Increases	Positive reinforcement	Negative reinforcement

Note: A behavior is something that is done. A stimulus is something in sensory impression (sight, sound, smell, feeling).

In **continuous reinforcement**, every response is followed by a reinforcement. This results in fast learning (acquisition) and results in fast extinction when reinforcement is stopped.

In **intermittent (or partial) reinforcement**, not every response is reinforced. Learning is slower and response is harder to extinguish; e.g., a child throws a tantrum and the parents ignore it for long periods of time in the hope that the child will stop. They don't want to reinforce such behavior with attention. However, if their patience wears thin and, after a long spell of ignoring, they attend to the baby, they are putting the child on an intermittent reinforcement schedule and will find it harder to extinguish the tantrums. Extinction of intermittent reinforcement often requires a change back to continuous reinforcement.

Interval schedules are based on the passage of time before reinforcement is given. A **fixed interval schedule** reinforces the response that occurs after a fixed period of time elapses. Responses are slow in the beginning of the interval and faster immediately prior to reinforcement.

- Response pattern: on and off
- Animal or person learns to delay response until near end of time period
- Cramming before an exam or working extra hard before bonus at the holidays

A **variable interval schedule** delivers reinforcements after unpredictable time periods elapse

- Higher, steadier rate of responding
- Cannot learn when next response will be reinforced, leading to a steadier response rate
- Pop quizzes or surprise bonuses at work

Ratio schedules are based on the number of behaviors elicited before reinforcement is given.

- **Fixed ratio schedule** delivers reinforcement after a fixed number of responses.
  - Produces high response rate
  - Rewards a set of behaviors rather than a single behavior, e.g., paying workers on a piecework basis.
- **Variable ratio schedule** delivers reinforcement after a changing number of responses.
  - Produces the greatest resistance to extinction
  - For example, in gambling, a large number of responses may be made without reward. Since any response may be the lucky one, person keeps on trying. Slot machines

Table 5-2. Reinforcement Schedules

		Contingency	
		Time	**Behaviors**
Schedule:	**Constant**	Fixed interval (FI)	Fixed ratio (FR)
	Changing	Variable interval (VI)	Variable ratio (VR)

Spontaneous recovery: after extinction, the response occurs again without any further reinforcement.

Secondary reinforcement: a symbol or a token gains reinforcement value because of its association with a real reinforcer (e.g., money is not valuable in itself but because of what you can do with it).

Modeling, Observational, or Social Learning

Watching someone else get reinforcement is enough to change behavior. This follows the same principles as in operant conditioning; correlating the effects of watching violence on television with committing violence "in the real world" stems from this concept and is part of why group therapy works. Other applications: assertiveness training, social skills training, preparing children for various frightening or painful medical or surgical procedures.

BEHAVIOR THERAPY AND BEHAVIOR MODIFICATION

Focus on treating symptoms directly rather than changing underlying internal conflicts.

Therapy/Modification Based on Classical Conditioning

Systematic desensitization usually begins with imagining oneself in a progression of fearful situations and using relaxation strategies that compete with anxiety. It is often used to treat anxiety and phobias and is based on the counterconditioning or reciprocal inhibition of anxiety responses.

- **Step 1:** Hierarchy of fear-eliciting stimuli is created, building from least to most stressful.
- **Step 2:** Therapist teaches the technique of muscle relaxation, a response that is incompatible with anxiety.
- **Step 3:** Patient is taught to relax in the presence, real or imagined, of each stimulus on the hierarchy from least to most stressful.

When the person is relaxed in the presence of the feared stimulus, objectively, there is no more phobia. Note that this works by replacing anxiety with relaxation, an incompatible response.

Via **exposure**, simple phobias can sometimes be treated by forced exposure to the feared object. Exposure is maintained until fear response is extinguished; e.g., a fear of heights is treated by having patient ride up elevator. More extreme form is called "flooding" or "implosion" therapy.

Aversive conditioning occurs when a stimulus that produces deviant behavior is paired with an aversive stimulus. Key properties of the original stimulus are changed; e.g., Pavlov's dog being presented with spoiled meat upon ringing bell. The dog does not salivate, but instead recoils as the spoiled meat is presented.

This is used in the treatment of alcoholism and some forms of sexual deviance; e.g., an alcoholic is given a nausea-inducing drug (disulfiram) whenever he drinks so that drinking eventually comes to elicit unpleasant rather than pleasant events; chili peppers and thumb-sucking.

Therapy/Modification Based on Operant Conditioning

Shaping (or successive approximations) achieves final target behavior by reinforcing successive approximations of the desired response. Reinforcement is gradually modified to move behaviors from the more general to the specific responses desired; e.g., an autistic boy who won't speak is first reinforced, perhaps with candy, for any utterance. From those utterances, the appropriate phonemes are selected and reinforced until the child utters the sought-after sounds. Eventually, reinforcement is contingent on his using speech correctly in the proper context.

Extinction involves discontinuing the reinforcement that is maintaining an undesired behavior; e.g., if complaining results in a patient receiving a lot of attention, stopping the attention will eventually stop the undesired behavior or instituting a "time out" with children who are acting inappropriately or test-takers who are anxious.

In **stimulus control**, sometimes stimuli inadvertently acquire control over behavior and when this is true, removal of that stimulus can extinguish the response; e.g., a person's eating behavior is tied to a particular stimulus, such as television watching, so reducing the time watching television should reduce the amount eaten or an insomniac is permitted in his bed only when he is so tired that he falls asleep almost at once.

Biofeedback (neurofeedback) uses external feedback to modify internal physiologic states. Certain functions of the autonomic nervous system (heart rate, blood pressure, body temperature) were once thought to be beyond the deliberate control of a person. We now know that both animals and humans can attain a measure of control over some bodily functions through the technique of biofeedback.

- Most biofeedback affects the parasympathetic system.
- Electronic devices present physiologic information, e.g., heart monitor to show heart rate, detailing one's internal responses to stimuli.
- Resulting trial-and-error learning requires repeated practice to be effective. Applications include treatment for hypertension, migraine and muscle-contraction headaches, Raynaud syndrome, torticollis, cardiac arrhythmias, and anxiety.
- Galvanic skin response: reduced skin conductivity = anxiety reduction

Fading is gradually removing the reinforcement without the subject discerning the difference; e.g., promoting smoking cessation by reducing the nicotine con tent of the cigarettes gradually and "silently" over a period of time or gradually replacing postoperative painkiller with a placebo.

Table 5-3. Learning-Based Therapies

Based on Classical Conditioning	
Systematic desensitization	Often used to treat anxiety and phobias **Step 1:** Hierarchy of stimuli: least to most feared. **Step 2:** Technique of muscle relaxation taught. **Step 3:** Patient relaxes in presence of each stimulus on the hierarchy. Works by replacing anxiety with relaxation, an incompatible response
Exposure (also: flooding or implosion)	Simple phobias treated by forced exposure to the feared object. Exposure maintained until fear response is extinguished
Aversive conditioning	Properties of the original stimulus are changed to produce an aversive response. Can help reduce deviant behaviors.
Based on Operant Conditioning	
Shaping	Achieves target behavior by reinforcing successive approximations of the desired response. Reinforcement gradually modified to move behaviors from general responses to the specific responses desired.
Extinction	Discontinuing the reinforcement that is maintaining an undesired behavior. "Time out" with children or for test-anxiety.

Based on Operant Conditioning	
Stimulus control	Sometimes stimuli inadvertently acquire control over behavior. When this is true, removal of that stimulus can extinguish the response. Example: an insomniac only permitted in bed when he/she is so tired that sleep comes almost at once.
Biofeedback	Using external feedback to modify internal physiologic states. Often uses electronic devices to present physiologic information, e.g., heart monitor to show heart rate. Works by means of trial-and-error learning and requires repeated practice to be effective.
Fading	Gradually removing the reinforcement: 1. without the subject discerning the difference 2. while maintaining the desired response Example: Gradually replacing postoperative painkiller with a placebo

Behavioral Models of Depression

Learned helplessness is a laboratory model of depression, where all normal avoidance responses are extinguished. If a rat is shocked and not allowed to escape, eventually, the rat will not take an obvious avoidance route even when it is offered.

Symptoms of helplessness in animals include passivity, norepinephrine depletion, and difficulty learning responses that produce relief, weight, and appetite loss. It is characterized in people by an attitude of "when nothing works, why bother." Increased levels of GABA in hippocampus decrease the likelihood of the learned helplessness response.

A low rate of response-contingent reinforcement is another explanation for depression. The person receives too little predictable positive reinforcement. A person may lack the social skills necessary to elicit this positive reinforcement. Depression can be seen as a prolonged extinction schedule; it results in passivity.

Review Questions

1. Psychiatric conditions must be understood as the result of biochemical imbalances and maladaptive behavioral patterns. The concept of "learned helplessness," important for the understanding of the behavioral patterns common in depressed patients, originates from animal studies in which the experimenter prevents

   A. spontaneous recovery
   B. extinction behavior
   C. stimulus generalization
   D. operant reinforcement
   E. avoidance behavior

2. At the direction of his parents, a child has learned to pick up his toys and clean his room each night before he goes to bed. To most increase the chances that the child will continue this behavior in the future, even when the parents are not present, continued reinforcement of the child should follow what type of reinforcement schedule?

   A. Fixed ratio reinforcement
   B. Fixed interval reinforcement
   C. Variable ratio reinforcement
   D. Variable interval reinforcement
   E. Noncontingent reinforcement

3. A child's crying can be the manifestation of an innate biological response or of conditioned behavior. Operant conditioning is most likely to account for which of the following instances of crying in an 18-month-old child? Crying that

   A. occurs spontaneously without any apparent cause
   B. increases in intensity when the adult does not respond
   C. occurs when the child is hungry
   D. occurs in response to an unexpected, sudden, painful stimulus
   E. occurs when the mother leaves the child in the care of a new babysitter

4. Two brothers have been fighting. Exasperated, the mother says to one of her sons, "Go to your room until you apologize to your brother for hitting him!" The mother's words are an example of the application of

   A. operant conditioning
   B. punishment
   C. aversive conditioning
   D. negative reinforcement
   E. extinction

5. After repeated exposure to a nurse in a white coat followed by an injection, a child learns to cower and cry in response to anyone approaching in a white coat. The child's behavior can best be explained as an example of

   A. shaping
   B. instrumental conditioning
   C. mediated reflex response arc
   D. classic conditioning
   E. observational learning

6. A man who has smoked 2 packs of cigarettes per day for 20 years decides to give up smoking, but is unsuccessful. When questioned by his physician, he notes that he has the most trouble refraining from smoking when he has his usual glass of bourbon every evening. Having "bourbon and a smoke" is how he relaxes at the end of the day. The physician suggests that he refrain from having bourbon each evening and substitute an evening stroll instead. The physician's advice is based on an application of the principle of

   A. aversive conditioning
   B. biofeedback
   C. systematic desensitization
   D. fading
   E. stimulus control

7. A 56-year-old man has just been diagnosed with diabetes. His physician is concerned about fostering adherence with a treatment regimen that includes regular medication and dietary changes. The patient will most likely follow instructions if the conversation with the physician makes the patient feel

   A. calm and collected
   B. calm and questioning
   C. concerned and attentive
   D. worried and distracted
   E. fearful and self-absorbed

Answers and Explanations

1. **Answer: E.** In the animal studies, the researcher prevents the animal from getting away from the painful stimulus: avoidance is prevented.

2. **Answer: C.** Variable ratio reinforcement is most resistant to extinction. Think of gambling.

3. **Answer: B.** Operant behavior is evident when an environmental stimulus, such as eye contact or the lack of response by the adult, evokes a learned behavior. Pain response is not learned, but innate.

4. **Answer: D.** The key here is the contingency; the child gets out of his room (removal of a stimuli) when he apologizes. This removal, making a behavior more likely, is the definition of negative reinforcement. Note, the mother's words are not punishment. That would be "you have been fighting with your brother, go to your room," trying to inflict punishment to limit a behavior.

5. **Answer: D.** White coat comes to be associated with pain, just as the bell comes to be associated with the meat for Pavlov. Classic, or its synonym, respondent conditioning.

6. **Answer: E.** By avoiding the stimulus that triggers the unwanted behavior, the unwanted behavior becomes less likely. Note that this is an application of operant conditioning.

7. **Answer: C.** The Health Belief model tells us that medium levels of anxiety are best for adherence.

Defense Mechanisms 6

Learning Objectives

- ❑ Use knowledge of 4 clusters of defenses
- ❑ Demonstrate understanding of transference

GENERAL ISSUES

Defense mechanisms are a concept born out of Freudian psychology. Recall that the Freudian psyche consists of:

- **Id:** animalistic, instinctive urges, sex, aggression, and other primary processes
- **Ego:** rational and language-based executors linking to reality
- **Super-ego:** the conscience, the moral compass insisting on socially acceptable behavior, sometimes to the point of individual deprivation begins to develop at age 5–9 (punitive)

Defenses are the primary tools of the ego, used to manage the internal conflicts between the primitive id and the punitive super-ego. They are the means by which the ego wards off anxiety and controls instinctive urges and unpleasant effects (emotions).

All defenses are unconscious, with one exception: **suppression**. Defenses change over time, and we are only aware of our defenses in retrospect. Defenses are adaptive as well as pathologic. We all use defenses all the time; they are how we cope.

Psychopathology is an issue of intensity and extent. Psychopathology = too much all at once, or for too extended a period of time. The key issue in psychopathology is the degree to which the use of defense mechanisms is disruptive of a person's ability to deal with the world around him or her. Unlike behaviorism, defenses are identified by what the person does in conjunction with his or her internal (unconscious) thought processes.

FOUR CLUSTERS OF DEFENSES

The clusters are presented from least mature to most mature.

Narcissistic Defenses

The boundary between self and others is highly permeable. One's sense of self is very weak and vulnerable.

Projection is when person attributes his own wishes, desires, thoughts, or emotions to someone else. Internal states are perceived as a part of someone else or of the world in general.

- A man who has committed adultery becomes convinced that his wife is having an affair even though there is no evidence of it
- A girl talks about her doll as having certain feelings, which are really what the girl feels
- A physician believes that the nursing staff is uncomfortable talking to him, when in fact, he is uncomfortable talking with them

Paranoia results from the use of projection.

Denial is not allowing reality to penetrate. Asserting that some clear feature of external reality is not true is used to avoid acknowledging of a painful aspect of reality.

- After surviving a heart attack, a patient insists on continuing his life-style as if nothing had happened
- A child who is abused insists that she has been treated well
- A woman prepares dinner for her husband expecting him to come home, even though he died a month earlier

Denial is often the first response to bad news, such as the impending death of a loved one or oneself. Substance users are often "in denial," claiming that they are not addicted and do not have a problem in the face of clearly dysfunctional or dangerous behavior.

Splitting is when people and things in the world are perceived as all bad or all good (God or the Devil). The world is pictured in extreme terms rather than a more realistic blend of good and bad qualities.

- "This doctor is a miracle worker, but that doctor is totally incompetent."
- "He's just so perfect and wonderful," says a teenage girl in love.
- "No one from that family will ever amount to anything; they are all just plain no good."

Borderline personality disorders use splitting and vacillate between seeing individuals in the world as all good or all bad. Prejudice and stereotypes are often the result of splitting.

Immature Defenses

The sense of self is stronger than with the narcissistic defenses, but the ego has areas of vulnerability.

Blocking is a temporary or transient block in thinking, or an inability to remember.

- "Mr. Jones, you are suffering from... gee, I just can't remember what it is called."
- A student is unable to recall the fact needed to answer the exam question, although he recalls it as he walks out of the exam.

- In the middle of a conversation, a woman pauses, looks confused, and asks what she was just talking about.

Blocking is disruptive and can be embarrassing.

Regression is returning to an earlier stage of development. "Acting childish" or at least younger than is typical for that individual.

- An older patient giggles uncontrollably or breaks down crying when told bad news.
- A husband speaks to his wife in "baby talk."
- A patient lies in bed curled up in a fetal position.

Play is regressive, i.e., a more free, simpler expression from a earlier age. Regression is common when people are tired, ill, or uncomfortable. **Enuresis** that develops in a child who previously had been continent following the birth of a new sibling is the result of regression. Similarly, when a new child is born, older children who have been weaned may demand to go back to breast-feeding.

During **somatization**, psychic derivatives are converted into bodily symptoms. Feelings manifest as physical symptoms rather than psychologic distress.

- Getting a headache while taking an exam
- Feeling queasy and nauseated before asking someone out on a date
- Developing a ringing in the ears while making a presentation for Grand Rounds

Extreme forms of somatization are diagnosed as somatic symptom disorders (see section on DSM-5). Symptoms created are physically real, not merely imagined

In **introjection** (identification), features of external world or persons are taken in and made part of the self. Introjection is the opposite of projection.

- A resident dresses and acts like the attending physician.
- A child scolds herself out loud in the same manner that her mother scolded her the day before.
- A teenager adopts the style and mannerisms of a rock star.

The superego is formed, in part, by the introjection of the same-gender parent as a resolution to the Oedipal crisis. Introjection is why children act like their parents. "I always swore that I would treat my children differently, yet there I was saying the same things to my children that my mother always used to say to me!" Being a sports fan or a soap opera fan involves introjection. Patients in psychotherapy gain a different (hopefully healthier) sense of self, in part, by introjecting their therapist.

Note

When identifying with others is done consciously, it is labeled "imitation."

Anxiety Defenses

Anxiety defenses serve to address the unpleasant discomforts of anxiety.

In **displacement**, the target of an emotion or drive changes, while the person having the feeling remains the same.

- A man who is angry at his boss pounds on his desk rather than telling his boss what he really thinks
- An attending physician scolds a resident who later expresses his anger by yelling at a medical student
- A married man who is sexually aroused by a woman he meets goes home and makes love to his wife

In family therapy, one child in the family is often singled out and blamed for all the family's problems, i.e., is treated as a scapegoat by others displacing their symptoms onto this child. Displacement often "runs downhill," i.e., from higher to lower in a power hierarchy. Phobias are the result of displacement.

In **repression**, an idea or feeling is eliminated from consciousness. Note that the content may once have been known, but now has become inaccessible.

- A child who was abused by her mother and was treated for the abuse, now has no memory of any mistreatment by her mother
- A man who survived 6 months in a concentration camp cannot recall anything about his life during that time period

In repression, you forget, and then forget that you forgot. Content is usually not recoverable without some trauma or psychoanalysis. Repression is differentiated from denial in that the reality was once accepted, but is now discarded. It is one of the most basic defense mechanisms.

In **isolation of affect**, reality is accepted, but without the expected human emotional response to that reality. There is separation of an idea from the affect that accompanies it.

- A child who has been beaten discusses the beatings without any display of emotions
- A physician informs a patient of his poor prognosis in bland, matter-of-fact tones
- A patient who severs his finger in an accident describes the incident to his physician with no emotional reaction

Isolation of affect involves facts without feelings. The bland affect of schizophrenics, *la belle indifference*, that often accompanies conversion disorder is a manifestation of this defense mechanism.

In **intellectualization**, affect is stripped away and replaced by an excessive use of intellectual processes. Cognition replaces affect. The intellectual content is academically, but not humanly, relevant.

- "Notice how the bone is protruding from my leg. It is interesting to contemplate the physics that allows such an event to happen."
- A physician tells a patient about his poor prognosis and discussed the technical aspects by which the prognosis was derived

- A boy who for the first time is about to ask a girl out talks with his friend about the importance of mating rituals for the long-term survival of the species and the mechanisms by which societies arrange for these rituals
- Intellect in place of emotion

Physicians who are too concerned with the technical aspects of the profession and not enough with the patient may well be using intellectualization. In obsessive–compulsive anxiety disorder, rumination can result from this defense mechanism.

Acting out is using a massive emotional or behavioral outburst to cover up underlying feeling or idea. Strong actions or emotions cover up unacceptable emotions. Note: The real emotion is covered, not expressed.

- Temper tantrum is thrown by an abandoned child to cover the depression he really feels
- "Whistling in the dark" hides the real underlying fear
- For adolescents, substance-related disorder, overeating, or getting into fights are "strong" actions that cover up underlying feelings of vulnerability

Acting out is differentiated from displacement in that the emotion is covered up, not redirected. It is common in borderline and antisocial personality disorders.

In **rationalization**, rational explanations are used to justify attitudes, beliefs, or behaviors that are unacceptable.

- "Yes, I believe killing is wrong, but I killed him because he really deserved it."
- A man who is unfaithful to his wife tells himself that this liaison will actually make him appreciate his wife more
- A young single woman tells herself that engaging in oral sex with a married man is not the same thing as having a "sexual relationship" with him

To identify, look for the "string of reasons." Note that this is not a reasoned action, but a search for reasons to allow an unacceptable action already selected. Rationalization is used to relieve guilt and shame and often accompanies obsessive–compulsive behavior.

In **reaction formation**, an unacceptable impulse is transformed into its opposite, for example, a global reversal in which love is expressed as hate.

- A student who always wanted to be a physician expresses relief and says, "This is the best news I've ever heard," after not being accepted into medical school.
- A teenage boy intrigued by "dirty pictures" organizes an anti-pornography campaign.
- Two coworkers fight all the time because they are actually very attracted to each other.

Excessive overreaction can be a sign of reaction formation, as if the person is trying to convince self, or anyone else, that the original feeling or impulse did not exist. From Shakespeare: "The lady doth protest too much, methinks." Found in many anxiety disorders.

Undoing is acting out the reverse of unacceptable behavior, as if to repair or fix the impulse.

- A man who is sexually aroused by a woman he meets immediately leaves and buys his wife flowers
- Superstitions such as "knock on wood" after wishing someone well
- A man repeatedly checks the burners on the stove to make sure that they are turned off before leaving the house

Many religions offer a type of institutionally sanctioned undoing: the penance after confession or making the sign of the cross to ward off anxiety. Obsessive–compulsive behavior (e.g., repeated hand-washing) is undoing.

Passive-aggression is nonperformance or poor performance after setting up the expectation of performance. Regarded as a passive (indirect) expression of hostility.

- "I could give you a good example of this, but I'm not going to."
- A student agrees to share class notes but goes home without sharing them
- A physician does not answer the direct questions of a patient whom he finds annoying

The feelings of hostility are unconscious, and the person using the defense is generally unaware of them. If you consciously set someone up, it is not a defense, but simply being mean. Often used by borderline personality disorders and young children.

Dissociation separates the self from one's experience. It is a third-person rather than first-person experience. The facts of the events are accepted, but the self is protected from the full impact of the experience.

- A woman who was raped reports that it was as if she was floating on the ceiling watching it happen
- The survivor of an automobile accident tells of the feeling that everything happened in slow motion
- A child who was sexually abused recalls only the bad man who came to her in her dreams

Dissociation is increasingly common in clinical settings. In extreme forms, it becomes a dissociative disorder, e.g., fugue states, amnesia, identity (multiple personality) disorder (see section on DSM 5).

Mature Defenses

Mature defenses distort reality less than the other defenses, and are thus considered more mature.

Humor permits the overt expression of feelings and thoughts without personal discomfort.

- A man laughs when told he is going to be fired
- A student smiles when he realizes that a particularly intimidating professor looks like a penguin
- A terminally ill cancer patient makes fun of his condition

Laughter covers the pain and anxiety. We laugh the easiest at the things that make us most anxious.

In **sublimation**, impulse gratification is achieved by channeling the unacceptable or unattainable impulse into a socially acceptable direction. The unacceptable/unattainable impulse becomes the motive force for social benefit.

- Dante wrote the *Inferno* as an outlet for his adoration of the woman Beatrice
- An executive who is attracted to a female associate becomes her mentor and advisor
- A patient with exhibitionist fantasies becomes a stripper

Much art and literature spring from sublimation, considered by some to be the most mature defense mechanism.

Suppression is the conscious decision to postpone attention to an impulse or conflict. Conscious setup and unconscious follow-through. The suppressed content temporarily resides in the unconscious.

- A student decides to forget about a pending exam to go out and have a good time for an evening
- A woman who is afraid of heights ignores the drop of the cliff to appreciate the beautiful vista
- A terminally ill cancer patient puts aside his anxiety and enjoys a family gathering

Unlike repression, suppressed content is recalled with the right cue or stimulus. Forget, but remember that you forgot.

TRANSFERENCE

The patient unconsciously transfers thoughts and feelings about a parent or significant other person onto his physician. This is not a defense mechanism. Transference can be positive (cause you to unaccountably like someone) or negative (cause you to unaccountably dislike someone).

- Easily established in cases of physical illness, because patient often undergoes a psychologic regression
- Not necessarily related to length of time the patient has known physician
- For a learning theorist, transference is just another instance of stimulus generalization
- Countertransference is transference from physician to patient

Table 6-1. Common Freudian Defense Mechanisms

Defense Mechanism	Short Definition	Important Associations
Projection	Seeing the inside in the outside	Paranoid behavior
Denial	Saying it is not so	Substance-related disorders, reaction to death
Splitting	The world composed of polar opposites	Borderline personality; good vs evil
Blocking	Transient inability to remember	Momentary lapse
Regression	Returning to an earlier stage of development	Enuresis, primitive behaviors
Somatization	Physical symptoms for psychological reasons	Somatic symptom disorders
Introjection	The outside becomes inside	Superego, being like parents
Displacement	Source stays the same, target changes	Redirected emotion, phobias, scapegoat
Repression	Forgetting so it is nonretrievable	Forget and forget
Isolation of affect	Facts without feeling	Blunted affect, *la belle indifference*
Intellectualization	Affect replaced by academic content	Academic, not human, reaction
Acting out	Affect covered up by excessive action or sensation	Substance-related disorders, fighting, gambling
Rationalization	Why the unacceptable is OK in this instance	Justification, string of reasons
Reaction formation	Unacceptable transformed into its opposite	Manifesting the opposite, feel love but show hate, "Girls have cooties"
Undoing	Action to symbolically reverse the unacceptable	Fixing or repairing, obsessive–compulsive behaviors
Passive-aggression	Passive nonperformance after promise	Unconscious, indirect hostility
Dissociation	Separating self from one's own experience	Fugue, depersonalization, amnesia, multiple personality
Humor	A pleasant release from anxiety	Laughter hides the pain
Sublimation	Unacceptable impulse into acceptable channel	Art, literature, mentoring
Suppression	Forgetting but it is retrievable	Forget and remember

Review Questions

1. "No, I don't remember, and I don't want to remember," cries a man asked to recall a painful episode from his childhood. The defense mechanism most closely suggested by this man's words and behavior is

   A. projection
   B. denial
   C. intellectualization
   D. dissociation
   E. repression

2. A woman finds herself in a town some distance from her home, without any recollection of how she got there. The defense mechanism that most likely accounts for this scenario is

   A. repression
   B. suppression
   C. dissociation
   D. reaction formation
   E. denial

3. When asked about his impending heart operation, the patient recounts the procedures in detail. He seems remarkably well versed and, upon questioning, admits that he has been "reading everything I can get my hands on" about it. He discusses the details for hours, yet shows no emotional reaction to the impending events. The defense mechanism that most likely accounts for this scenario is

   A. rationalization
   B. repression
   C. regression
   D. isolation
   E. intellectualization

4. A woman with no previous history of promiscuity suddenly begins to take on sexual partners of both sexes, one right after the other. The record shows that her new pattern of sexual behavior started soon after the death of a child to whom she was very close. Yet, there is no indication of a period of mourning. The woman's behavior suggests the defense mechanism of

   A. isolation
   B. suppression
   C. denial
   D. acting out
   E. undoing

5. A 32-year-old Irish male appears at the clinic complaining of "a slight pain" on his left side. Upon examination, he is found to have two broken ribs. When informed of this, the man insists that it cannot be that serious and asks only for some medication for the pain. This is best characterized as the defense mechanism of

   A. displacement
   B. denial
   C. depression
   D. isolation
   E. reaction formation

6. A father, who has lost his daughter as the result of a traffic accident involving a drunk driver, organizes a local chapter of a national group campaigning to stop the sale of liquor to minors and to legislate mandatory jail time for anyone convicted of drunk driving. "If I can't have my girl back, at least I can make sure it doesn't happen to some other father," he says. The defense mechanism that most likely accounts for this behavior is

   A. acting out
   B. suppression
   C. reaction formation
   D. displacement
   E. sublimation

7. A 64-year-old factory worker is hospitalized after barely surviving a serious myocardial infarction. His life was saved by the administration of emergency balloon angioplasty. The following day, his primary care physician visits the patient's hospital room. Much to his surprise, he finds the patient, who never did much exercise before, on the floor doing push-ups and saying, "Time to get in shape, doc!" The patient's word and behavior in this instance are most likely the result of the defense mechanism of

   A. denial
   B. dissociation
   C. acting out
   D. undoing
   E. reaction formation

8. Bob is an avid sports fan who runs 5 miles everyday for fitness and relaxation, and frequently plays touch football with others in this neighborhood. One day after he had had an argument with his wife, Bob got into a fistfight during a football game and had to be restrained by his teammates. The defense mechanism that most likely accounts for Bob's behavior is

   A. acting out
   B. denial
   C. displacement
   D. dissociation
   E. intellectualization
   F. introjection
   G. isolation
   H. passive–aggression
   I. projection
   J. rationalization
   K. reaction formation
   L. regression
   M. repression
   N. splitting

Answers and Explanations

1. **Answer: E.** Repression is forgetting, and forgetting that you forgot. It is enduring and motivated by unconscious desires. Repression is one of the most basic defense mechanisms.

2. **Answer: C.** Amnesia with travel is the classic definition of psychogenic fugue state, the result of dissociation as a defense mechanism.

3. **Answer: E.** Rather than responding with the expected level of apprehension and anxiety, the patient spends his time reading and cognitive activity. Anxiety is replaced by cognitive activity: intellectualization.

4. **Answer: D.** Rather than showing the expected grief reactions, the woman embarks on a new course of behavior. This behavior masks the underlying, unexpressed feeling and constitutes acting out.

5. **Answer: B.** The patient responds to the reality of broken ribs by saying that it is not so. This bald-faced negation of objective facts is denial.

6. **Answer: E.** The father gets gratification from the impulse to save his daughter by helping others. The behavior is not simply redirected as with displacement, but targeted directly to the issue of concern to the benefit of others.

7. **Answer: D.** The patient is acting to fix or make up for his heart condition. This behaviorally focused reversal is what undoing is all about.

8. **Answer: C.** The anger Bob feels toward his wife is redirected into a fight with someone else. Bob is still angry, but the recipient of the anger changes from his wife to another.

Psychologic Health and Testing 7

Learning Objectives

- ❑ Differentiate between psychologic health and physical health
- ❑ Demonstrate understanding of intelligence quotient (IQ)
- ❑ List commonly used personality tests
- ❑ Demonstrate understanding of neuropsychologic tests

PSYCHOLOGIC HEALTH AND PHYSICAL HEALTH

Type A behavior pattern (or the coronary prone behavior pattern) is a cluster of behavioral traits that has been associated with increased prevalence and incidence of coronary heart disease. The extreme Type A person is engaged in a chronic struggle to obtain an unlimited number of things from his environment in the shortest possible period of time. He tends to be impatient, competitive, preoccupied with deadlines, and highly involved with his job.

Recent data suggest that how people handle hostility is the key component of Type A behavior. People who get hostile and angry at everyday slights are more at risk. One major prospective study has shown that the Type A behavior pattern is associated with a twofold increase in incidence of coronary heart disease, even after controlling for the major risk factors (systolic blood pressure, cigarette smoking, cholesterol). Following a first heart attack, Type As who survived had a lower chance of a second attack than did Type Bs.

PSYCHOLOGIC ADJUSTMENT AND PHYSICAL HEALTH

A study of physically healthy men (Harvard sophomores between 1942 and 1944) followed for nearly 40 years showed that mentally healthy individuals do not deteriorate in physical health as quickly as do those in poor mental health. Chronic anxiety, depression, and emotional maladjustment predict negative health events later in life.

Holmes and Rahe scale is used to quantify stressful life events. On this scale, different life events contribute different weightings to the total score. The death of a spouse is weighed as the most stressful event. The correlation between stressful life events and developing illness is a small but significant positive correlation between +0.30 and +0.40.

Individuals react differently to the same objective stressors due to the individual's appraisal of the meaning of the stressor and Hardy personality type: clear sense of values, goals, and capabilities; an unshakable sense of the meaningfulness of life; and a strong sense of control over one's own fate.

Social support: Belief is more important than objective support. Having one significant person to turn to is key. Women use support more effectively than do men. Presence of a familiar person lowers blood pressure in a person under stress. Widows and widowers have higher rates of heart attacks in the year just after a spouse dies.

Physiologic changes in response to stress include key stress response pathway: hypothalamic-pituitary-adrenal axis; cortisol levels rise then fall within 24 hours after stressor; secondary spike in cortisol levels 48 to 72 hours after stressor.

INTELLIGENCE QUOTIENT (IQ)

IQ is a general estimate of the functional capacities of a person; 70% inherited, recent studies suggest most from mother. IQ is not an absolute score but a comparison among people. Distribution mean: 100; standard deviation: 15.

Table 7-1. Distribution of IQ Scores in the General Population

Range	Label	Distribution
Less than 69	Intellectual disability	About 2.5% of the population
70 to 79	Borderline	
80 to 89	Low average	
90 to 109	Average	About 50% of the population
110 to 119	High average	
120 to 129	Superior	
over 130	Very superior	About 2.5% of the population

Calculating an intelligence quotient by mental age method:

- Mental age (MA) = median test score for a given age
- Chronological age (CA) = actual age of the person taking the test
- Formula: $\frac{MA}{CA} \times 100 = \text{IQ score}$

Example: A 10-year-old child got a test score of 25. If 25 is the median score of 13-year-olds, then MA = 13, CA = 10, and $\frac{13}{10} \times 100 = 130$ Note that as CA goes up, if MA stays constant, IQ goes down.

Calculating an IQ by deviation from norms method:

- For each age range (cohort), take a sample of the IQ test scores.
- The mean is 100 and the standard deviation is 15.
- If a child age 10 scores a 25 on the test, find the table for age 10 and look up a score of 25 to see what IQ level the score corresponds to

Error margin for both mental age method and deviation from norms method is ±5 points.

IQ is highly correlated with education and is an excellent predictor of academic achievement. Mental illness is distributed across all ranges of intelligence, although measured IQ may be lower when assessed because of interference of symptoms.

Autistic children tend to be of below-average intelligence, with 80% having IQs less than 70.

Longitudinal tests for intelligence show very little decline in the elderly; verbal ability holds up best, while perceptual and motor tests show some decline.

IQ is very stable from age 5 onward; increased exposure to verbal behavior early in life leads to a higher IQ.

IQ tests contain elements of cultural bias, asking about words and objects more familiar in some cultures than in others.

Commonly used IQ tests:

- Wechsler Adult Intelligence Scale, Revised (WAIS-R) is for adults, aged 17 and older.
- Wechsler Intelligence Scale for Children, Revised (WISC-R) is for children aged 6 to 17.
- Wechsler Preschool and Primary Scale of Intelligence (WPPSI) is for children aged 4 to 6.
- Stanford-Binet Scale was the first formal IQ test (1905) and is used for children aged 2 to 18. Today, it is most useful with children younger than 6, the impaired, or the very bright.

PERSONALITY TESTS

Objective tests: simple stimuli (usually questions), restricted range of responses possible (select between choices given), scored mechanistically using scoring key; no clinical experience required to score. There are 2 types of objective personality test:

- **Criterion referenced:** results are given meaning by comparing them with a preset standard, e.g., "Every student who scores above 75% will pass."
- **Norm referenced:** results are given meaning by comparing them with a normative group. Classic example is Minnesota Multiphasic Personality Inventory (MMPI) revised 1989:

- >550 statements to which respondent answers true or false
- Most widely used (and misused) personality test. Serves as criterion for newly developed tests
- Yields 10 primary clinical dimensions and 3 validity scales

Projective tests: ambiguous stimuli; wide range of responses possible, scored by experienced clinician using consensual standards. Meaning of responses found by clinical correlation between collected cases of responses and personal characteristics, psychopathologies.

- Rorschach Inkblot Test: Patients are asked to look at an inkblot and report what they see.
- Thematic Aperception Test (TAT): Patients are asked to tell a story about what is going on in the pictures.
- Sentence Completion Test: Patient is asked to complete a set of sentence stems with the first thing that comes to mind.
- Projective drawings: Patient is given a sheet of paper and asked to draw a house, a tree, a person, a family, or some other subject.

NEUROPSYCHOLOGIC TESTS

Halstead-Reitan Battery: Tests for presence and localization of brain dysfunction. Consists of 5 basic tests: category test, tactual performance test, rhythm test, speech sounds perception test, finger oscillation test. These are combined to provide an impairment index.

Luria Nebraska Battery: Tests level of impairment and functioning. Subscales: motor, rhythm, tactile, visual–spatial, receptive speech, expressive speech, writing, reading, arithmetic, amnestic, intellectual, right and left hemisphere function.

Bender Visual Motor Gestalt Test: Screens for brain dysfunction. Nine designs are presented to the patient and copied by him. The patient is then asked to recall as many designs as he or she can.

Benton Visual Retention Test: Spatial construction, drawing task. 10 designs that the patient copies as presented or from memory.

Wechsler Memory Scale: Assesses memory impairment. Subcomponents: recall of current and past information, orientation, attention, concentration, memory for story details, memory designs, and learning. Yields a memory quotient.

Human Development 8

Learning Objectives

- ❑ Use knowledge of developmental milestones to determine if a child is developmentally delayed
- ❑ Demonstrate understanding of applying child-development principles
- ❑ List warning signs of child abuse

DEVELOPMENTAL MILESTONES

General Patterns in Human Development

Development occurs along multiple lines: physical, cognitive, intellectual, and social. We tend to chart development for each of these lines in terms of milestones, i.e., skills achieved by a certain age. Milestones are simply normative markers at median ages. Some children develop slower and some faster. The ages for the milestones are therefore only approximate and should not be taken as dogma. Although children generally progress along the lines of development together, they often may not. Thus, a child may match the milestones for cognitive development but show slower growth in the social area.

Infants

Recent research has changed our past assumptions about the capabilities of infants. Evidenced at birth:

- Reaching and grasping behavior
- Ability to imitate facial expressions
- Ability to synchronize their limb movements with speech of others (coupling or entrainment)
- Attachment behaviors, such as crying and clinging

Newborn preferences:

- Large, bright objects with lots of contrast
- Moving objects
- Curves versus lines
- Complex versus simple designs
- Evidence of a preference for facial stimuli

The fact that a neonate will demonstrate defensive movements if an object looms toward her face suggests that she can perceive a 3-dimensional world.

Recent research also suggests that the neonatal nervous system gives special attention to language versus nonlanguage stimuli. Left-brain–evoked potentials are larger than right-brain–evoked potentials to language stimuli (but not to nonlanguage stimuli). Neonates can discriminate between language and nonlanguage stimuli. Infants do not learn language but learn to use the language capacity they are born with (Broca's area).

At just 1 week old, the infant responds differently to the smell of the mother compared with the father.

The smile develops from an innate reflex present at birth (endogenous smile). An infant shows exogenous smiling in response to a face at 8 weeks. A preferential social smile, e.g., to the mother's rather than another's face, appears about 12 to 16 weeks.

Physical development. Hands and feet are the first parts of the body to reach adult size. Motor development follows set patterns:

- Grasp precedes release
- Palm up maneuvers occur before palm down maneuvers
- Proximal to distal progression
- Ulnar to radial progression
- Capacity to copy shapes follows in alphabetical order: circle, cross, rectangle, square, triangle. The exception is a "diamond," which can generally not be reproduced until age 7.
- First words (10 months), then first birthday, then first steps (13 months)

Figure Copied	Approximate Age
Circle	3
Cross	4
Rectangle	4½
Square	5
Triangle	6
Diamond	7

Figure 8-1. Figures Copied and Approximate Ages

A **brain-growth spurt** is the "critical period" of great vulnerability to environmental influence; extends from last trimester of pregnancy through first 14 postnatal months. The size of cortical cells and complexity of cell interconnections undergo their most rapid increase. The brain adapts structure to match environmental stimulation.

- Earliest memories, roughly ages 2–4
- Stranger anxiety: distress in the presence of unfamiliar people; appears at 6 months, reaches its peak at 8 months, disappears after 12 months; can occur even when child is held by parent

Separation anxiety is infant distress following separation from a caretaker; appears at 8–12 months; begins to disappear at 20–24 months. Continued separation, especially prior to 12 months, leads to withdrawal and risk of anaclitic depression. School phobia (Separation Anxiety Disorder) is failure to resolve separation anxiety. Treatment focuses on child's interaction with parents, not on activities in school.

Imprinting is an interesting facet of attachment behavior in animals. Some animals (geese, ducks, quail) will follow the first object they see after birth; may even run to it, rather than to the mother, when frightened. Imprinting does not apply to humans.

Table 8-1. Child Development Milestones

Age	Physical and Motor Developments	Social Developments	Cognitive Developments (Piaget)	Language Developments
1st year of life	• Puts everything in mouth • Sits with support (4 mo) • Stands with help (8 mo) • Crawls, fear of falling (9 mo) • Pincer grasp (10 mo) • Follows objects to midline (4 wk) • One-handed approach/grasp of toy • Feet in mouth (5 mo) • Bang and rattle stage • Changes hands with toy (6 mo)	• Parental figure central • Issues of trust are key • Stranger anxiety (7 mo) • Play is solitary and exploratory • Pat-a-cake, peek-a boo (10 mo)	• Sensation/movement • Schemas • Assimilation and accommodation	• Laughs aloud (4 mo) • Repetitive responding (8 mo) • "ma-ma, da-da" (10 mo)

Age	Physical and Motor Developments	Social Developments	Cognitive Developments (Piaget)	Language Developments
Age 1	• Walks alone (13 mo) • Climbs stairs alone (18 mo) • Emergence of hand preference (18 mo) • Kicks ball, throws ball • Pats pictures in book • Stacks 3 cubes (18 mo)	• Separation anxiety (12 mo) • Dependency on parental figure (rapprochement) • Onlooker play	• Achieves object permanence	• Great variation in timing of language development • Uses 10 words
Age 2	• High activity level • Walks backwards • Can turn doorknob, unscrew jar lid • Scribbles with crayon • Stacks 6 cubes (24 mo) • Stands on tiptoes (30 mo) • Able to aim thrown ball	• Selfish and selfcentered • Imitates mannerisms and activities • May be aggressive • Recognizes self in mirror • "No" is favorite word • Parallel play	• A world of objects • Can use symbols • Transition objects • Strong egocentrism • Concrete use of objects	• Use of pronouns • Parents understand most • Telegraphic sentences • Two-word sentences • Uses 250 words • Identifies body parts by pointing
Age 3	• Rides tricycle • Stacks 9 cubes (36 mo.) • Alternates feet going up stairs • Bowel and bladder control (toilet training) • Draws recognizable figures • Catches ball with arms • Cuts paper with scissors • Unbuttons buttons	• Fixed gender identity • Sex-specific play • Understands "taking turns" • Knows sex and full name		• Complete sentences • Uses 900 words • Understands 4 × that • Strangers can understand • Recognizes common objects in pictures • Can answer, "Tell me what we wear on our feet?" • "Which block is bigger?"
Age 4	• Alternates feet going down stairs • Hops on one foot • Grooms self (brushes teeth) • Counts fingers on hand	• Imitation of adult roles • Curiosity about sex (playing doctor) • Nightmares and monster fears • Imaginary friends	• Points to and counts 3 objects • Repeats 4 digits • Names colors	• Can tell stories • Uses prepositions • Uses plurals • Compound sentences

Age	Physical and Motor Developments	Social Developments	Cognitive Developments (Piaget)	Language Developments
Age 5	• Complete sphincter control • Brain at 75% of adult weight • Draws recognizable man with head, body, and limbs • Dresses and undresses self • Catches ball with 2 hands	• Conformity to peers important • Romantic feeling for others • Oedipal phase	• Counts 10 objects correctly	• Asks the meaning of words • Abstract words elusive
Ages 6 to 12	• Boys heavier than girls • Permanent teeth (11 y) • Refined motor skills • Rides bicycle • Prints letters • Gains athletic skill • Coordination increases	• "Rules of the Game" are key • Organized sport possible • Being team member focal for many • Separation of the sexes • Sexual feelings not apparent • Demonstrating competence is key	• Abstract from objects • Law of conservation acheived • Adherence to logic • Seriation • No hypotheticals • Mnemonic strategies • Personal sense of right and wrong	• Shift from egocentric to social speech • Incomplete sentences decline • Vocabulary expands geometrically (50,000 words by age 12)
Age 12 + (adolescence)	• Adolescent "growth spurt" (girls before boys) • Onset of sexual maturity (10+ y) • Development of primary and secondary sexual characteristics	• Identity is critical issue • Conformity most important (11–12 y) • Organized sports diminish for many • Cross-gender relationships	• Abstract from abstractions • Systematic problemsolving strategies • Can handle hypotheticals • Deals with past, present, future	• Adopts personal speech patterns • Communication becomes focus of relationships

Table 8-2. Tanner Stages (Pubic Hair)

Look for	Median ages
1. No hair	$\leq$ 10 years
2. Small amount, downy	10 to 11 years
3. Hair coarse and curly	11 to 13 years
4. Adult-like but not on thigh	13 to 14 years
5. Extends to medial thigh	> 14 years

APPLYING CHILD-DEVELOPMENT PRINCIPLES

Discipline of Children

Be sure discipline is developmentally age-appropriate. Abstract, cognitive reasonings mean little to a child younger than 6 years. If trying to stop a young child from hitting another, don't expect the child to understand how the other feels. Best application of discipline would be "time out." Punishment by hitting the child is too confusing; you are doing exactly what you are telling the child not to do. Discipline should be clearly connected (in time and space) to behavior to be modified.

Teenagers

Identity formation is the key issue; issues of independence and self-definition predominate. The teenage years may be stressful but are not generally filled with the type of traumas often portrayed in the popular press. Teenagers' values reflect those of their parents. Rebellion is manifested as minor disagreements regarding hair, music, dress, friends; most likely in early teenage years. Sexual experimentation with opposite- and same-sex partners is common.

Attachment and Loss

In childhood: Bowlby postulates 3 phases of response to prolonged separation of children aged 7 months to 5 years:

- Protest: crying, alarm, aggression
- Despair: hopes of regaining loved one fades
- Detachment: feelings of yearning and anger are repressed

Psychologic upset is more easily reversed in stages of protest or despair than after detachment has set in. Because separation has behavioral consequences, pediatric hospitalization must take it into account through provision of parental contact (e.g., rooming-in practices, flexible visiting hours, assurances that mother will be present when child awakes from surgery).

In adults: Adults who are bereaved or are mourning the loss of a loved one also go through a series of phases.

- Initial phase (protest, acute disbelief): lasts several weeks, weeping, hostility and protest

- Intermediate phase (grief, disorganization): 3 weeks to 1 year; sadness, yearning, somatic symptoms; obsessional review, searching for deceased; may believe they see or hear deceased; confronting reality
- Recovery (or reorganization) phase: reinvestment of energies and interests; begins second year after death, memories fade in intensity

Table 8-3. Normal Grief versus Depression

Normal Grief	Depression
Normal up to 1 year	After 1 year, sooner if symptoms severe
Crying, decreased libido, weight loss, insomnia	Same but more severe
Longing, wish to see loved one, may think they hear or see loved one in a crowd (illusion)	Abnormal overidentification, personality change
Loss of other	Loss of self
Suicidal ideation is rare	Suicidal ideation is common
Self-limited, usually less than 6 months	Symptoms do not stop (may persist for years)
Antidepressants not helpful	Antidepressants helpful

Dealing with Dying Patients

People move back and forth through the stages of adjustment (Kubler-Ross). Not everyone passes through all stages or reaches adequate adjustment. The stages do not have to occur in order.

- Denial
- Anger
- Bargaining
- Depression
- Acceptance

The stages are similar for dealing with loss or separation. Rules for dealing with the dying:

- Tell the patient everything.
- Do not give false hope.
- Allow person to talk about feelings.
- Keep involved in activities.
- Avoid social isolation.

Children's Conceptions of Illness and Death

Children do not see the real world, do not live in the same world that we do. They have a limited cognitive repertoire; their thinking is concrete and egocentric. When they become ill, they may interpret this as a punishment and may have misconceptions about what is wrong with them.

Children from birth to 5 years old really have no conception of death as an irreversible process. More than death, the preschool child is more likely to fear separation from parents, punishment, mutilation (Freud's castration anxiety). Only after age 8 or 9 is there understanding of the universality, inevitability, and irreversibility of death.

Facts about the Elderly and Aging

In the United States, the fastest growing age cohort is people age >85. The. U.S. population age ≥65 was 4% in 1960, 11.2% in 1980, and 13% in 2010.

The elderly account for over 35% of all health care expenditures. Roughly 70% of men age >75 are married, but only 22% of women. Around 13% of the elderly are below the poverty line, which is the same rate as that of the total population. (The rate is 2x greater for Hispanics and 3x greater for blacks.)

Only 5–10% of those age >65 have moderate or severe dementia. For those age >85, the rate is 25%. Half of dementia cases are due to Alzheimer's disease.

With the exception of cognitive impairment, the elderly have a **lower incidence** of all psychiatric disorders compared with younger adults. Preventive occupational therapy (OT) programs offer clear advantages over "just keeping busy" to reduce decline in mental and physical health in the elderly.

The elderly in the United States are generally not isolated or lonely, but may not receive the same respect as in other cultures. The family is still the major social support system for the elderly in times of illness; 80% have children and most have frequent contact with them. Institutionalization is undertaken only as a last resort.

The best predictor of nursing home admissions is falls and fall-related injuries. Exercise will improve an elderly person's balance and help reduce the risk of falls. Also, "safe proofing" the home will help.

- 85% of the elderly have at least 1 chronic illness, and half have some limitation to their activities.
- Only 5% are homebound.
- About 2 million, or about 6% are institutionalized; among the noninstitutionalized, 60% call their health excellent or good, 20% fair.
- One in 10 persons age ≥75 is in a nursing home; for those ≥85, the ratio is 1 in 5.

ABUSE

Child Abuse

More than 6,000 children are killed by parents or caretakers each year in the United States. More than 3 million annually are reported abused, with half confirmed by investigation. Many abuse cases likely go unreported.

Abuse is defined by:

- Tissue damage
- Neglect

- Sexual exploitation
- Mental cruelty

Abuse is a mandatory reportable offense up to age 18. Failure to do so is a criminal offense. If case is reported in error, the physician is protected from legal liability. Remember it is your duty to protect the child (separate from the parents), as well as your duty to report.

Clinical signs:

- Broken bones in first year of life
- Sexually transmitted disease (STD) in young children
- 92% of injuries are soft tissue injuries (bruises, burns, lacerations).
- 5% have no physical signs.
- Nonaccidental burns have a particularly poor prognosis. They are associated with death or foster home placement. If burn is on arms and hands, it was likely an accident; if burn is on arms but not hands, it is more likely abuse.
- Shaken baby syndrome: look for broken blood vessels in eyes

Children at risk for abuse are:

- Younger than 1 year of age
- Stepchildren
- Premature children
- Very active
- "Defective" children

Parents are likely themselves to have been abused, and/or perceive child as ungrateful and as cause of their problems.

Be careful not to mistake benign cultural practices such as "coining" or "moxibustion" as child abuse; these and other folk medicine practices should usually be accepted. Key is whether practice causes enduring pain or long-term damage to child. Treat female circumcision as abuse. Look for an opening to discuss with parents how they treated child prior to seeing the physician.

Children who are abused are more likely to:

- Be aggressive in the classroom
- Perceive others as hostile
- View aggression as a good way to solve problems
- Have abnormally high rate of withdrawal (girls)
- Be unpopular with school peers and other children; the friends they do have tend to be younger.

Child Sexual Abuse

Each year, 150,000 to 200,000 cases of sexual abuse are reported. 50% of sexual abuse cases are within the family; 60% of victims are female. Most victims are aged 9 to 12 years; 25% of victims younger than 8 years. Most likely source: uncles and older siblings, although stepfathers are also more likely. In general, males more likely to be sources.

Risk factors:

- Single-parent families
- Marital conflict
- History of physical abuse
- Social isolation

More than 25% of adult women report being sexually abused as a child (defined as sex experience before age 18 with a person 5 years older): 50% by family members; 50% told no one. Sexually abused women are more likely to:

- Have more sexual partners
- Have 3–4× more learning disabilities
- Have 2× more pelvic pain and inflammation
- Be overweight (slight increased risk)

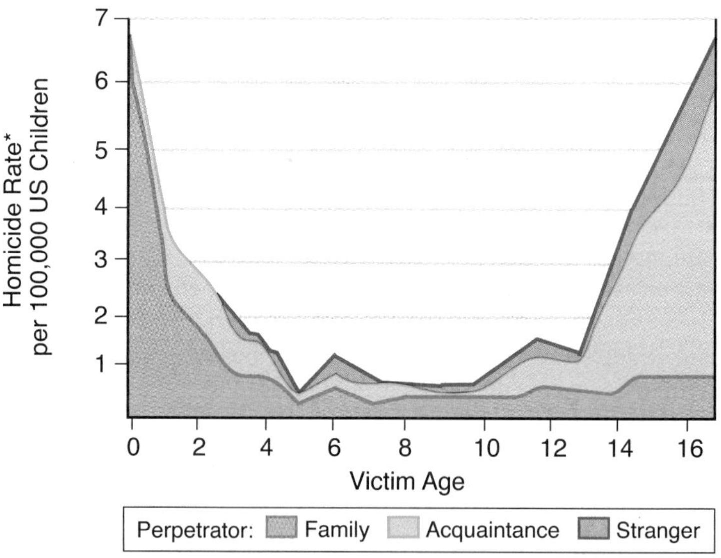

Figure 8-2. Relationship of Child Homicide Victims to Perpetrators

Domestic Partner Abuse

An estimated 4 to 6 million women are beaten each year. Each year, 1,500 women are killed by their abusers. Not mandatory reportable offense. If confronted with a case, give the victim information about local shelters and counseling.

- Number of attacks has held steady since mid-1970s.
- Domestic violence is the #1 cause of injury to American women (for men, traffic accidents and other unintentional injuries are #1).
- Occurs in all racial and religious backgrounds, and across all SES groups
- More frequent in families with drug abuse, especially alcoholism
- If one attack occurs, more are likely.

Male more likely abuser if he considers his wife his belonging, is jealous or possessive, and there are verbal assaults to his self-esteem.

Female more likely abused if she grew up in a violent home (about 50%), married at a young age, perceives self as unable to function alone (dependent), is pregnant, last trimester (highest risk).

Abused spouses tend to blame themselves for the abuse, identification with the aggressor.

Elder Abuse

Elder abuse is a mandatory reportable offense with a prevalence rate 5 to 10%. Includes physical, psychological, financial, or neglect; neglect is the most common type (50% of all reported cases). Caretaker is the most likely source of abuse; spouses are often caretakers.

Table 8-4. Types of Abuse and Important Issues

	Child Abuse	Elder Abuse	Domestic Abuse
Annual cases	Over 2 million	5 to 10% in population	Over 4 million
Most common type	Physical battery/neglect	Neglect	Physical battery
Likely gender of victim	Before age 5: female After age 5: male	63% Female	Female
Likely gender of perpetrator	Female	Male or Female	Male
Mandatory reportable?	Yes	Yes	No
Physician's response	Protect and report	Protect and report	Counseling and information

Review Questions

1. An 8-year-old girl attains a score of 35 on a standard intelligence test. Included in the test-scoring packet is a table showing median test scores for specific ages. An extract from the table is presented below:

Age	Median Score
4	15
5	18
6	22
7	25
8	29
9	32
10	35
11	40
12	45

Based on this table, the most likely IQ for this 8-year-old girl is

A. 85
B. 100
C. 110
D. 125
E. 140

2. A psychiatric researcher develops an observational test to assess the level of impulse control found in bipolar patients. As a part of the test development strategy, the results of this observational test are compared with patients' scores on a standard paper-and-pencil test that also assesses impulse control. If the observational test has a high correlation with the paper-and-pencil test, the researcher would be most likely to regard this as evidence for

A. construct validity
B. test-retest reliability
C. predictive validity
D. split-half reliability
E. convergent validity

3. A 55-year-old executive makes a habit of doing several things at once. He always seems to be in a hurry and frequently worries that there are just not enough hours in the day to get things done. He is impatient with his subordinates and often gets angry with them when they do not perform to his standards or get their work to him on time. The pattern of behavior displayed by this man suggests that in the next 10 years he is most at risk for developing

    A. a gastric ulcer
    B. prostate cancer
    C. respiratory difficulties
    D. mental health problems
    E. an acute myocardial event

4. A 5-year-old child is referred to a mental health practitioner for evaluation. The practitioner wants to gain insight into the conscious and unconscious preoccupations of the child. To accomplish this objective, the practitioner is most likely to make use of

    A. Luria Nebraska Battery
    B. Halsted-Reitan Battery
    C. Minnesota Multiphasic Personality Inventory
    D. Projective Drawing Test
    E. Rorschach test
    F. Wechsler Intelligence Scale for Children

5. A 3-year-old boy talks when his parents are talking in spite of being repeatedly told not to do so. His parents become frustrated with his behavior and ask his physician about the reason for this behavior pattern. The physician should advise the parents that this tendency of children to test the extremes of behavior that their parents will tolerate

    A. is indicative of later maladjustment
    B. persists with partial parental reinforcement
    C. results from the action of classic conditioning
    D. can be resolved by a clear, reasoned explanation to the child
    E. is more commonly observed in boys than girls

6. A 5-month-old and a 12-month-old infant observe their mothers leaving the room. Which one will most likely begin to cry?

    A. The 5-month-old
    B. The 12-month-old
    C. Both will cry
    D. Neither will cry

7. A young child is able to walk when held by one hand and speaks in strings of unrecognizable words. When placed in a room with other children, the child stays close to his mother but plays by himself. Based on these observations, in the next 6–8 months the child is most likely to learn to

   A. ride a tricycle
   B. stand on his tiptoes
   C. draw a circle
   D. build a tower of 3 blocks
   E. play peek-a-boo

8. A child is observed walking down the stairs using alternating feet, can throw and catch a ball, states her gender accurately, and is able to correctly name the colors of presented objects. Based on this evidence, which of the following geometric shapes did the child most recently learn to draw?

   A. Cross
   B. Diamond
   C. Square
   D. Triangle
   E. Circle

9. Conformity with peers is a core characteristic of a number of normative developmental stages. In general, conformity of children to the norms of their peer groups is most intense at a time of development that also features

   A. toilet training
   B. use of transition objects
   C. focal attachment to the caretaker
   D. beginning of formal schooling
   E. puberty

10. Studies of infants in wartime and natural disasters have revealed a number of characteristic changes in the expected developmental sequence. In comparison with those undergoing normal development, infants who experience severe psychosocial deprivation are more likely to display

   A. separation anxiety
   B. infantile symbiosis
   C. anxiety with strangers
   D. delayed language development
   E. rapprochement

11. Although much of human behavior is learned, infants are born with certain capacities. Which of the following important behavioral skills are present in most infants at birth?

    A. Following objects to midline
    B. Laughing aloud
    C. Putting feet into mouth
    D. Reaching and grasping
    E. Recognition of the mother

12. A 4-year-old girl is brought by her mother to see the local pediatrician. The mother insists that the girl be given a complete physical exam. The physical exam turns up nothing abnormal. The mother insists that something must be wrong with the girl because she spends hours playing by herself and talking with a "friend" that no one else can see. In addition, 2–3 times a week the girl wakes up screaming from nightmares and is convinced that there is some sort of "monster" in her closet that is going to eat her as she sleeps. The physician's next action should be to

    A. ask the mother about any recent trauma or changes in the girl's life
    B. reassure the mother that the girl is displaying normal behavior for her age
    C. re-examine the girl for signs of sexual abuse
    D. schedule the girl for psychiatric evaluation
    E. send the girl for a neurologic consultation

13. An 8-year-old girl is brought to the emergency department by her grandmother, who reports that she found the girl sitting in her apartment, dirty and disheveled, during a heat wave. The girl reports that she had not eaten in 2 days or seen her mother in the past 24 hours. Physical examination shows the girl to be severely dehydrated and lethargic in her responses to physical stimuli. At this point, the physician's next step would be to

    A. ask the girl if she would like to stay in the hospital for a while
    B. contact the local child welfare agency
    C. contact the police and report the girl's mother for neglect
    D. initiate IV fluids for the child
    E. obtain permission from the grandmother to begin treatment for the child
    F. try to contact the girl's mother

14. A 67-year-old woman visits her physician 4 months after the death of her husband. She reports that she has difficulty sleeping and often finds herself crying at the "smallest things." The physician notices that she has lost weight and seems to avoid eye contact when interviewed. With some embarrassment, she confesses that she came to see the physician after thinking that she saw her husband across the street in a crowd, an experience that left her confused and shaken. At this point, the physician's best response would be to

    A. ask her if she has much interest in sex lately
    B. ask her to talk about her relationship with her husband prior to his death
    C. detain her for observation as a suicide precaution
    D. explain to her that she has an adjustment disorder
    E. schedule her for a psychiatric evaluation
    F. tell her that these are normal reactions and that adjustment takes time
    G. write her a prescription for antidepressants

Answers and Explanations

1. **Answer: D.** Use the mental age method. (MA/CA) × 100 = IQ score. A score of 35 is median for a 10-year-old. Therefore, (10/8) × 100 = 125

2. **Answer: E.** Reliability means consistency. Validity means detecting truth. When two similar tests produce the same result, we have a confirmation of truth called convergent validity.

3. **Answer: E.** The question presents an example of type A behavior pattern. People who display this behavior pattern are more than 2x as likely to experience a heart attack.

4. **Answer: D.** The limited verbal skills of the child make this the best choice. Note that the Wechsler is an IQ test that does not give the information sought. The Halsted-Reitan and Luria Nebraska are batteries which assess and localize brain dysfunction.

5. **Answer: B.** Children will always learn by testing. This is normal behavior and not indicative of maladjustment. However, it persists, like any behavior, if the parents reinforce it even unintentionally.

6. **Answer: B.** The key issue here is the timing of separation anxiety. It begins between 8 to 12 months of age and continues for most of the second year of life. The 5-month-old is too young. The 12-month-old is in the right age range.

7. **Answer: D.** The child described is about age 1 year. Stacking 3 blocks is expected by about age 18 months. The child should already know peek-a-boo, standing on tiptoes is achieved at about age 30 months, riding tricycle and drawing a circle are skills learned at about age 3 years.

8. **Answer: A.** The child described is about age 4 years and has most recently learned to draw a cross. Circle is age 3 years, and square is age 5 years. The other options are for age 6 and up.

9. **Answer: E.** Conformity is most intense between ages 11 and 13, although it is also important during ages 4 to 6.

10. **Answer: D.** All of these listed are part of normal development with the exception of delayed language development. Infantile symbiosis is part of the early attachment relationship between mother and child. Rapprochement occurs as the child is learning separation from the parents.

11. **Answer: D.** Following objects to midline is 4 weeks, feet in mouth and laughing aloud about 4 to 5 months. It takes the infant about a week after birth before it can recognize the mother.

12. **Answer: B.** Imaginary friends and nightmares are common in children of this age. They represent normal developmental patterns and are NOT indicative of abuse, trauma, or more deep-seated psychological problems.

13. **Answer: D.** This victim of child neglect requires essential medical intervention. Care for the patient's needs first, and then worry about contacting the appropriate child welfare agency.

14. **Answer: F.** The question portrays a woman in normal grief, both by description and time frame. She needs reassurance that her reactions, including "seeing" her husband, are a part of a normal grief process.

9 Sleep and Sleep Disorders

Learning Objectives

- ❑ Demonstrate understanding of sleep architecture
- ❑ Explain information related to developmental aspects of sleep
- ❑ Answer questions about biochemistry of sleep
- ❑ Describe common sleep disorders

SLEEP ARCHITECTURE

Sleep consists of 2 distinct states: NREM and REM.

Non–Rapid Eye Movement Sleep (NREM)

NREM is divided into 4 stages on the basis of EEG criteria. It alternates with REM sleep throughout the sleep period and is characterized by:

- Slowing of the EEG rhythms
- Higher muscle tone
- Absence of eye movements
- Absence of "thoughtlike" mental activity

NREM is an idling brain in a movable body.

Rapid Eye Movement Sleep (REM)

REM is an awake brain in a paralyzed body. It is characterized by:

- An aroused EEG pattern
- Sexual arousal
- Saccadic eye movements
- Elaborate visual imagery (dreaming)
- Associated with pons

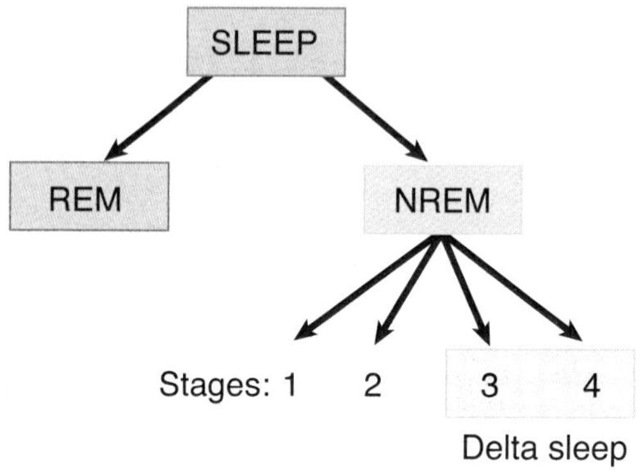

Figure 9-1. Types of Sleep

Biologic Rhythms

The sleep-wake cycle itself is a circadian rhythm, i.e., an endogenous cyclic change occurs in an organism with a periodicity of roughly 24 hours. The cycle is regulated by the superchiasmatic nucleus (SCN). The REM cycle, which is ~90 minutes, is an example of an ultradian rhythm, occurring with a periodicity of <24 hours.

Sleep Facts

Most of NREM stages 3 and 4 (the deepest sleep levels) occur during the first half of the night; together, stages 3 and 4 are called delta sleep or slow-wave sleep.

Most REM sleep occurs during the last half of the night; REM sleep gets progressively longer as the night goes on.

The average adult spends most sleep time in stage 2, and least time in stage 1. Adults most commonly wake out of REM or stage 2 sleep. The duration of one's delta sleep is 65% inherited.

Latency

Sleep latency is the period between awake until sleep onset; typically 5–15 minutes. Insomniacs have long sleep latency.

REM latency is the period between falling asleep until first REM. In the average adult, REM latency is 90 minutes.

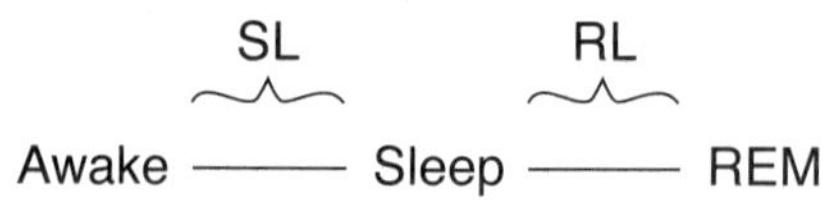

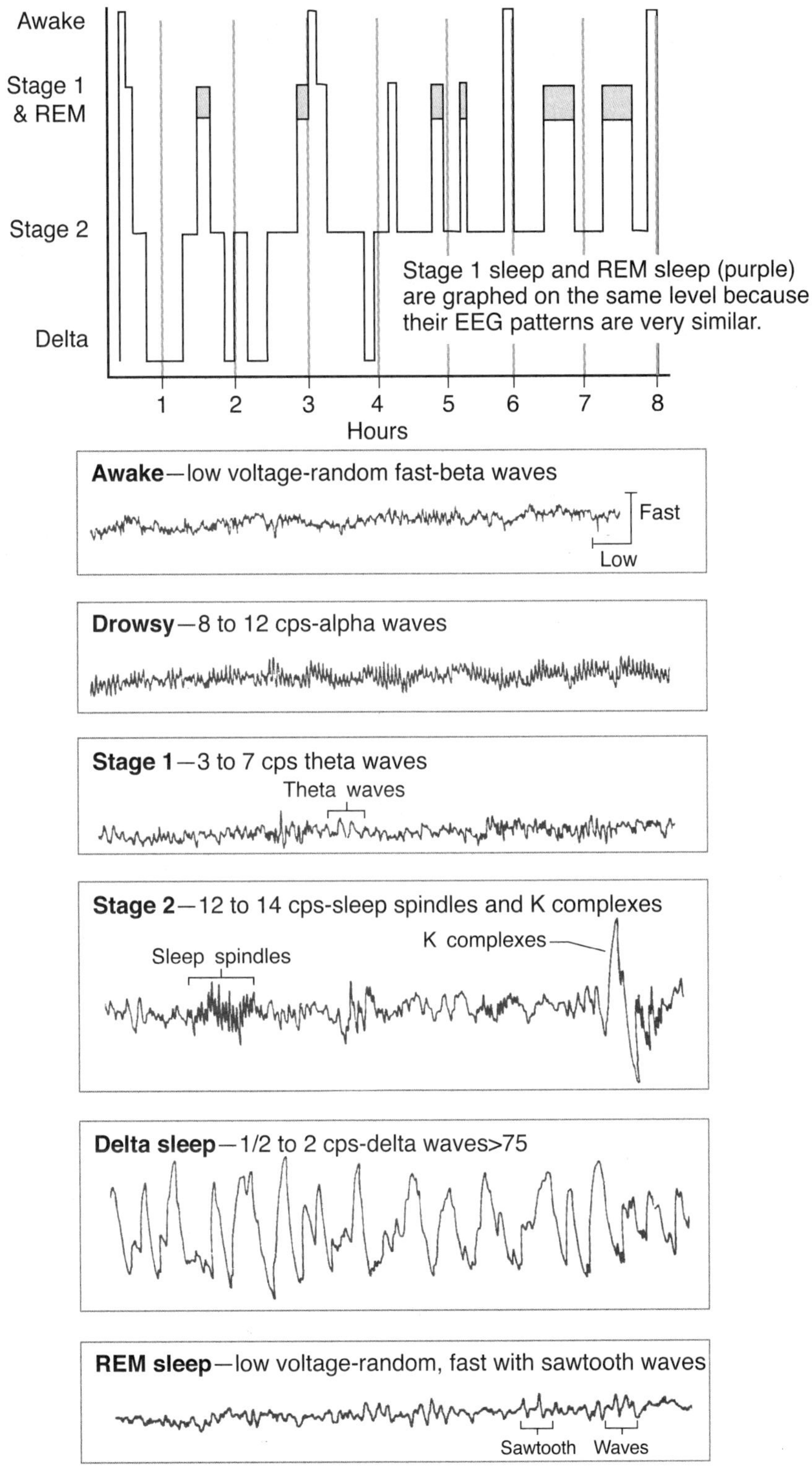

Figure 9-2. Sleep Architecture Diagram Showing Stages of Sleep in Sequence

Sleep Deprivation

The cerebral cortex shows the greatest effects of sleep deprivation but has the capacity to cope with one night's sleep loss. The rest of the body seems relatively unaffected by sleep deprivation. Physical restitution of the body comes from the immobility that is a by-product of sleep, not from sleep itself.

Only about 35% of lost sleep is made up: ~80% of lost stage 4 is recovered and 50% of missing REM is recovered.

- If one gets ≤5 hours of sleep per night, functioning will be at the level of someone legally drunk!
- The longer the prior period of wakefulness, the more Stage 4 sleep increases during the first part of the night and the more REM declines.
- Short sleepers lose the latter part of REM sleep.

In sleep-deprived individuals, the following occurs:

- Lymphocyte levels decline
- Cortisol levels rise
- Blood pressure rises
- Glucose tolerance is reduced
- Greater amygdala activation
- Lower prefrontal cortical activity
- Increased negative mood

REM sleep appears to increase somewhat in both children and adults after learning, especially the learning of complex material in the previous waking period. REM sleep is essential to get the most out of studying, as that is when most long-term memories are consolidated by the hippocampus.

REM deprivation does not impede the performance of simple tasks. It does, however, interfere with the performance of more complex tasks, make it more difficult to learn complex tasks, and decrease attention to detail (though not the capacity to deal with crisis situations). Delta sleep increases after exercise and seems to be the result of raised cerebral temperature.

Table 9-1. Changes in First 3 Hours of Sleep

Human growth hormone (HGH)	Increase
Prolactin	Increase
Dopamine	Decrease
Serotonin	Increase
Thyroid-stimulating hormone (TSH)	Decrease

Melatonin is not related to sleeping, but rather to feelings of sleepiness. It is produced in the pineal gland and directly in the retina of the eyes.

- Sensitive to light via a pathway from the eyes
- Release is inhibited by daylight, and, at nighttime, levels rise dramatically

- Likely mechanism by which light and dark regulate circadian rhythm
- Responsible for "jet lag"
- Responsible for seasonal affective disorder (SAD)
- Adjust melatonin with bright light therapy, not pills

DEVELOPMENTAL ASPECTS OF SLEEP

Sleep develops during childhood and adolescence into adult patterns.

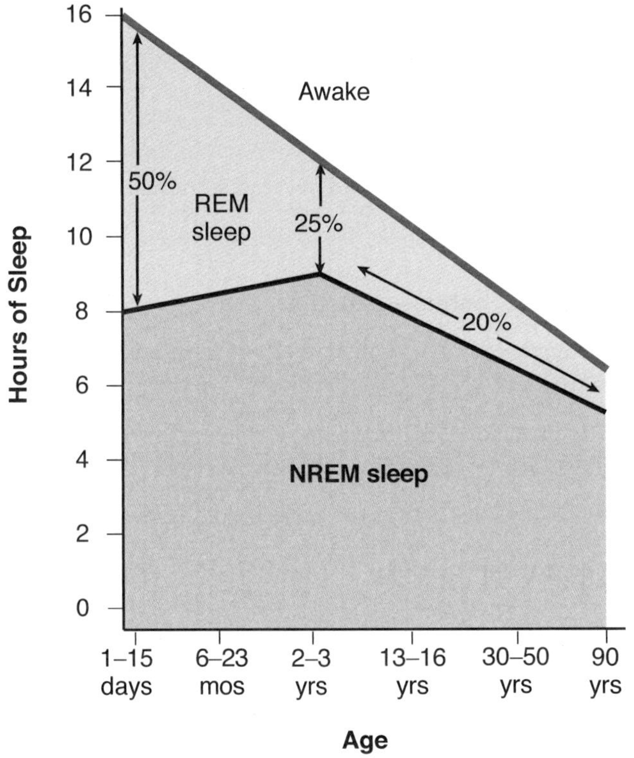

Figure 9-3. Changes in Daily Sleep Over the Life Cycle

Age	Total Sleep Time/24 Hours
Neonate	16–18 hours
1 y	12 hours
10 y	10 hours
13–16 y	8 hours

Age	Number of Sleep Periods/24 Hours
Neonate	6–9
1–2 y	2–3
5–10 y	1

Sleep patterns of **infants**:

- Premature infants do not demonstrate a discernible sleep-wake cycle.
- By about age 1 year, EEG demonstrates adult-like rhythms of sleep and wakefulness.
- Neonatal sleep cycle starts at 30–40 min and gradually lengthens to 90 min by teens
- Mismatch of infant and adult cycles produces "sleep fragmentation" for new parents

Sleep patterns of **adults**:

- Initial REM cycle is approximately 90 min; subsequent cycles throughout evening are shorter
- REM: 20% of sleep time
- Total sleep time/24-hour period decreases gradually with age.

Sleep patterns of **elderly**:

- Total sleep time continues to decline.
- REM percentage remains constant (20%) until around age 80, then declines further
- Stage 4, then stage 3 NREM (delta sleep) vanish; elderly often complain they feel less rested than they used to

BIOCHEMISTRY OF SLEEP

Chemical and Psychiatric Correlates of Sleep

Any pharmacology that increases **dopamine** increases wakefulness. Dopamine blockers (e.g., antipsychotics) increase sleep somewhat.

Benzodiazepines cause limited decrease in REM and Stage 4 sleep, much less than previously thought. There is little rebound effect. Chronic use increases sleep latency.

Moderate **alcohol consumption** leads to early sleep onset and increased wakefulness during the second half of the night. **Intoxication** decreases REM; REM rebound (with nightmares) occurs during withdrawal.

Barbiturates decreases REM; REM rebound, including nightmares, follows stoppage of chronic use.

Major depression increases REM, decreases REM latency (45 rather than 90 minutes), and decreases Stages 4 and 3 sleep. It leads to increased sleep in multiple periods over 24 hours, early morning waking, diurnal improvement. Sleep deprivation gives 60% remission from symptoms. People who characteristically get a lot of REM are more susceptible to onset of depression.

Neurotransmitters Associated with Sleep: "SANDman"

Serotonin: helps initiate sleep

Acetylcholine (ACh): higher during REM sleep (associated with erections in men)

Norepinephrine (NE): lower during REM sleep

- Ratio of ACh and NE is the biochemical trigger for REM sleep.
- NE pathway begins in the pons, which regulates REM sleep.

Dopamine: produces arousal and wakefulness. Rises with waking

SLEEP DISORDERS

Narcolepsy

Narcolepsy is a condition characterized by the brain's inability to control sleep-wake cycle. The narcoleptic tetrad:

- Sleep attacks and excessive daytime sleepiness (EDS)
- Cataplexy (pathognomonic sign)
- Hypnagogic hallucinations (hypnopompic can occur, but not pathognomonic): hypnagogic is while falling asleep and hypnopompic is while waking up
- Sleep paralysis

Narcolepsy is a disorder of REM sleep: onset of REM within 10 minutes. Linked to deficiency in hypocretin when cataplexy is present. Loss of hypocretin results in an inability to regulate sleep.

Treatment:

- Modafinil or psychostimulants for EDS: inhibits DA re-uptake; activates glutamate; inhibits GABA
- Antidepressants (TCA, SNRI)
- Gamma hydroxybutyrate (GHB) to reduce daytime sleepiness and cataplexy

Types of **sleep apnea** include obstructive or upper airway sleep apnea (middle-aged, overweight, rasping snoring), central or diaphragmatic sleep apnea (elderly, overweight, Cheyne-Stokes–60-second hyperventilation, followed by apnea), and mixed sleep apnea.

Clinical presentation and features include

- High risk of sudden death during sleep, development of severe nocturnal hypoxemia, pulmonary and systemic hypertension (with elevated diastolic pressure)
- Nocturnal cardiac arrhythmias (potentially life-threatening)
- Bradycardia, then tachycardia

- Males outnumber females by 8 to 1
- EDS and insomnia often reported
- Heavy snoring with frequent pauses
- Kicking, punching of sleeping partner
- Obesity is often part of the clinical picture, but not always
- Short sleep duration, frequent waking, insomnia, decreased Stage 1, decreased delta and REM

Treatment:

- Weight loss (if applicable)
- Behavioral conditioning to change sleep position
- Continuous positive airway pressure (CPAP) most likely medical intervention
- For severe obstructive and mixed apnea: tonsillectomy or tracheostomy

Sudden Infant Death Syndrome (SIDS): Unexplained Death in Children Age <1

SIDS causes 3,000 deaths annually; 50% reduction in incidence if baby placed on back, rather than on stomach. Avoid overstuffed toys and pillows. Rate is 2–3 × times higher in families where someone smokes. 5-HT levels 26% below normal. Fetal exposure to maternal smoking also a strong risk factor.

Insomnia

Secondary to hypnotic medication abuse; development of tolerance to sedative hypnotics is common and leads to escalating doses. Sleep architecture becomes disrupted and sleep fragmentation occurs.

Other possible causes: emotional problems, especially anxiety, depression, mania; conditioned poor sleep, sleep cycle is so disrupted that habit of sleep is lost; withdrawal from drugs or alcohol.

When working up an insomniac, examine for medical explanations such as apnea and drug use (prescription or illicit), as well as psychiatric factors such as depression, anxiety, and schizophrenia. 50% of insomnia in sleep labs is due to psychological factors. Insomniacs may have GABA levels 30% lower than normal.

Treatment:

- Sleep hygiene
- Behavior therapy still is best (most effective): muscle relaxation and stimulus control
- Drugs: action on GABA receptors (zaleplon, zolpidem, eszopiclone); ramelteon (melatonin receptor agonist (MT1, MT2); low chance of dependence; no hangover or rebound)

Night Terrors versus Nightmares

Table 9-2. Differences Between Night Terrors and Nightmares

	Night Terrors	Nightmares
Sleep stage	Stage 4 (delta sleep)	REM
Physiologic arousal	Extreme	Elevated
Recall upon waking	No	Yes
Waking time anxiety	Yes, usually unidentified	Yes, often unidentified
Other issues	Runs in families More common in boys Can be a precursor to temporal lobe epilepsy	Common from ages 3 to 7 If chronic, likelihood of serious pathology Desensitization behavior therapy provides marked improvement

Note

Research suggests that getting an extra 30–40 minutes of sleep a night greatly reduces both nightmares and night terrors.

Somnambulism (Sleep-Walking)

Occurs in the first third of the night. Stage 4 sleep (Delta). If wakened, the person is confused and disoriented. Treat with benzodiazepines.

Enuresis (Bed-Wetting)

Most seen in stages 3 and 4 sleep, but can occur in all stages. Boys 2× as likely as girls. At age 5, 7% of boys, 3% of girls. Boys cease wetting later. Often history with same-sex parent. Common after change or new sibling born; defense mechanism of regression. Treat with desmopressin, imipramine, or bell pad technique.

Bruxism (Teeth-Grinding)

Occurs during stage 2 sleep. Prevention is to use oral device to prevent teeth grinding.

10 Physician-Patient Relationship

Learning Objectives

- ❑ Demonstrate understanding of general rules of the physician-patient relationship

The physician-patient relationship is a potent healing partnership based on trust. In the setting of a productive alliance there are tremendous opportunities for clinical interventions that can significantly improve the patient's health and quality of life. The key is what the ideal physician should do.

Rule #1: The patient is number one.
Always place the interests of the patient first. Choose the patient's comfort and safety over yours or anyone else's. The goal is to serve the patient, not to worry about legal protection for the physician. Make it a point to ask about and know the patient's wishes.

Rule #2: Nothing should be between you and patient.
Get rid of tables and computers.; if you must have a table, pick the smallest one. Ask family members to leave the room; if the patient requests that they stay, then that is okay.

Rule #3: Tell the patient everything, even if you have not been asked.
Answer any question that is asked of you. Respond to the emotional as well as the factual content of questions. The patient should know what you know, and as soon as you know it; if you have only partial information, say that it is partial and tell what you know. Do not force a patient to hear bad news if he does not want it at that moment, but do try to discuss it with him as soon as possible. We tell them so they tell us; make reciprocity the norm. Information should flow through the patient to the family, not the reverse.

Rule #4: Work on a long-term relationship, not just short-term problems.
Each encounter is an opportunity to develop a better relationship. Make eye contact. Practice defined touch: tell her what you are doing. Arrange seating for comfortable, close communication; sit so you are at the same eye level if possible.

Rule #5: Listening is better than talking.
Be an "information sponge." You know what matters, but the patient won't. Getting the patient to talk is generally better than having you talk. Ask what the patient knows before explaining. Take time to listen, even if other patients or colleagues are waiting. End the encounter by asking, "Is there anything else?" Allow silences while patients search for words.

Rule #6: Negotiate rather than order.
Treatment choices are the result of agreement, not commands by the physician. Remember, the patient makes medical decisions from the choices provided by the physician. Relationship and agreement support adherence.

Rule #7: Solve the problem presented.
Look for a "solution," not the "answer." Stay in the room; do not leave. Change your plan to deal with new information when it is presented. Don't assume that the patient likes or trusts you. Treat difficult or suspicious patients in a friendly, open manner.

Rule #8: Admit to the patient when you make a mistake.
Everything is your responsibility. Take responsibility; don't blame it on the nursing staff or on a medical student. Admit the mistake even if it was corrected and the patient is fine.

Rule #9: Never "pass off" your patient to someone else.
Refer to a specialist when something is beyond your expertise (but this is usually not the case). Refer only for ophthalmology or related subspecialties. You provide instruction in aspects of care, e.g., nutrition, use of medications.

Rule #10: Express empathy, then give control.
When faced with a patient who is grieving or angry or when faced with upset family members, first acknowledge and legitimize their feelings. "I'm sorry, what would you like to do?"

Rule #11: Agree on the problem before moving to a solution.
Discuss the diagnosis fully before moving to treatment options. Ask what a patient knows about the diagnosis before explaining it. Tell him your perceptions and conclusions about the condition before moving to treatment recommendations. Informed consent requires the patient to fully understand what is wrong. Offering a correct treatment before the patient understands his condition is wrong.

Rule #12: Be sure you understand what the patient is talking about before intervening.
Patients may present problems with much emotion without clearly presenting what they are upset about. Seek information before acting; when presented with a problem, get some details before offering a solution. Begin with open-ended questions, then move to closed-ended questions.

Rule #13: Patients do not get to select inappropriate treatments.
Patients select treatments, but only from presented, appropriate choices. If a patient asks for an inappropriate medication that she heard advertised, explain why it is not indicated. Make conversations positive. Talk about options that are available; don't just say no to a patient's request.

Rule #14: Best answers serve multiple goals.
Think broadly about everything you want to achieve. Consider both short- and long-term goals. Best answers deal with patients' health issues, while supporting relationships and acting ethically.

Rule # 15: Never lie.
There is no such thing as a "white lie." Do not lie to patients, their families, or insurance companies. Do not deceive to protect a colleague.

Rule #16: Accept the health beliefs of patients.
Be accepting of benign 'folk medicine' practices. Expect them. Diagnoses need to be explained in the way patients can understand, even if not technically precise. Offer to explain things to family members.

Rule #17: Accept patients' religious beliefs and participate if possible.
Your goal is to make the patient comfortable. Religion is a source of comfort to many. A growing body of research suggests that patients who pray and are prayed for have better outcomes. Ask about a patient's religions beliefs if you are not sure (but not as a prelude to passing off to the chaplain!). Of course, you are not expected to do anything against your own religious or moral beliefs, or anything which risks patient's health.

Rule #18: Anything that increases communication is good.
Take the time to talk with patients, even if others are waiting. Ask "why?" Ask about the patient beyond the disease: job, family, children. Be available. Take calls. Answer emails.

Rule #19: Be an advocate for the patient.
Work to get the patient what she needs. Never refuse to treat a patient because she cannot pay.

Rule #20: The key is not so much what you do, but how you do it.
Focus on the process, not just goals; focus on means, not just ends. Do the right thing, the right way. The right choices are those that are humane and sensitive, and put the interests of the patient first. Treat family members with courtesy and tact, but the wishes and interests of the patient come first.

MISCELLANEOUS PHYSICIAN-PATIENT RELATIONSHIP TOPICS

The key is not the amount of time spent with a patient, but what is done during that time. Lack of rapport is the chief reason that terminally ill patients reject medical advice, or why patients change physicians or miss appointments. Failure of patient to cooperate, or even to keep appointments, should be seen as the result of physician insensitivity or seeming indifference.

An early Scandinavian study found a significant increase in sudden deaths on a coronary care unit during or immediately following ward rounds. The formality of rounds and the imposing authority that physicians project onto patients may have raised patient anxiety to dangerous levels.

The amount of information that surgical candidates receive about their upcoming operation and about the postsurgical pain affects outcome. Patients given more information about what to anticipate were ready for discharge 2.7 days earlier than were controls. They also requested 50% less morphine.

A good rapport fosters adherence to treatment regimens and is positively associated with a reduction of malpractice suits.

Asking Questions of the Patient

An **open-ended question** allows broad range for answer. A **closed-ended question** limits answer, e.g., yes or no. A **leading question** suggests or indicates preferred answer.

- **Confrontation:** brings to the patient's attention some aspect of appearance or demeanor
- **Facilitation:** gets the patient to continue a thought, talk more, "tell me about that..."
- **Redirection:** puts question back to the patient
- **Direct question:** seeks information directly. Avoid judgmental terms.

Fostering Patient Adherence

It is not enough for a physician to provide information and treatment and leave adherence to the patient. The physician must present information in ways that will optimize patient adherence.

Patients are less compliant when limited information has been exchanged and when there is dissatisfaction with the interview. A consistent complaint is that insufficient medical information was made available to the patient (or to the parents). Fewer positive statements made by the physician and less sought-after information offered by the physician results in less patient compliance.

For best adherence:

- Attend to the amount of information
- Explain its complexity
- Note the patient's affective state
- Explain why this particular treatment is being recommended

- Stress the threat to health of nonadherence
- Stress the effectiveness of the prescribed regimen
- Give instructions both orally and in writing
- Arrange for periodic follow-up
- Ask patient to do less

Research has shown that physicians cannot tell which of their patients do and do not adhere. They assume that more of their patients are adhering than actually are. When a patient does fail to adhere, do not blame the patient. If the patient is nonadherent, check for these problems:

- Patient dissatisfaction with the physician
- Misunderstanding of instructions
- Interference by family
- Inability to afford medications

The health belief model states adherence is a function of perceived threat and moderate fear level is best for adherence. Recall the curvilinear relationship between fear and adherence. Perceived threat is a function of perceived seriousness and perceived susceptibility. External barriers, such as finances or lack of access to care, can prevent adherence even if perceived threat is sufficient.

Review Questions

1. Psychiatric diagnoses and exogenous pharmacology have long been associated with specific changes in sleep patterns. Based on current sleep laboratory data, decreases in rapid eye movement sleep would most likely occur in a patient who has been

   A. abusing alcohol
   B. taking L-tryptophan purchased at a health food store
   C. diagnosed with a major affective disorder
   D. taking lithium carbonate
   E. diagnosed with a generalized anxiety disorder

2. A 35-year-old woman complains that she has trouble sleeping at night. Her physician prescribes a course of benzodiazapines to deal with this problem. As he hands her the prescription, he should also caution her that prolonged use of this class of medications to induce sleep will most likely result in the appearance of what side effect?

   A. Sleep apnea syndrome
   B. Depressed mood
   C. Insomnia
   D. Nocturnal enuresis
   E. Somnambulism

3. At about the same time that children are toilet trained, their sleep patterns are characterized by

   A. about 50% of time in REM
   B. 2–3 sleep periods throughout the day
   C. about 15 hours of total sleep time per day
   D. achievement of the 90-minute sleep cycle
   E. initiation of Stage 4 sleep

4. K-complexes are characteristic of a stage of sleep also distinguished by

   A. delta waves
   B. theta waves
   C. sawtooth waves
   D. alpha waves
   E. sleep spindles

5. In a typical 30-year-old adult, the first 3 hours of sleep each night are accompanied by a measurable increase in

   A. corticosteroids
   B. output of human growth hormone
   C. dopamine
   D. thyroid-stimulating hormone
   E. norepinephrine

6. A measurable increase in delta stage sleep is often observed following

   A. alcohol intoxication
   B. ingestion of melatonin
   C. medication with imipramine
   D. onset of major depression
   E. physical exercise

7. A 45-year-old male presents to his physician complaining of fatigue. He reports difficulty going to sleep each night, waking up multiple times each night, and headache upon awaking in the morning. His wife has started sleeping on the couch because of his loud snoring and thrashing during the night. Physical exam shows the patient to be 40 pounds overweight and hypertensive. Based on this preliminary information, the physician suspects that the most likely underlying cause of the patient's reported problems is

   A. bruxism
   B. central apnea
   C. insomnia
   D. narcolepsy
   E. nightmares
   F. night terrors
   G. obstructive apnea
   H. restless legs syndrome

8. A 35-year-old woman goes to see a gynecologist for her first visit on a hot August day. The physician walks into the examination room to find the woman still fully dressed, fidgeting in her chair, and looking around the examination room nervously. The physician introduces himself and shakes the patient's hand. The patient's hand is sweating and clammy. At this point, what should the physician say next?

   A. "Boy, it sure is hot out today."
   B. "Don't worry. I have been doing this for years."
   C. "Is something wrong?"
   D. "I need you to get undressed so we can get started."
   E. "Let me tell you about my credentials and training."
   F. "So what brings you in here today?"
   G. "This is our first meeting. Tell me a little bit about yourself."
   H. "You need to relax. I won't hurt you."
   I. "You seem a little nervous. That's normal at this point."

9. Following an annual physical exam, a 43-year-old woman asks her physician for a prescription to cope with anxiety. When the physician points out she has no symptoms and has never mentioned the need before, the woman confesses that the prescription is for her husband who works during normal office hours and is unavailable to come make the request himself. The physician's best response would be

   A. give her the prescription, but ask that her husband schedule an appointment as soon as possible
   B. give her the prescription, but instruct her that she should give her husband the medication only if he really needs it
   C. give her a referral for her husband to a local psychiatrist
   D. offer to write her husband a prescription if he will call and talk with you on the phone
   E. offer to write her husband the prescription after he comes in for a scheduled appointment
   F. refuse to write the prescription
   G. tell her that you will see her husband outside of normal office hours and evaluate the need for the prescription

10. A 68-year-old woman, referred by a health management organization (HMO), complains angrily to her physician about how long she had to wait before he was able to see her. The physician's best response would be

   A. "I'll speak to the receptionist."
   B. "I'm very sorry you had to wait so long. How can we do better in the future?"
   C. "It will never happen again."
   D. "Please understand my staff is very busy."
   E. "Things just take longer with these HMOs."
   F. "Well, you are here now. What can I do for you?"
   G. "Would you like to come back on another day?"

11. A mother takes her 2-year-old boy who is suffering from severe diarrhea to see the pediatrician. Stool samples reveal the presence of *Campylobacter jejuni*. At this point, what is the next action the physician should take?

    A. Describe to the boy's mother the dangers inherent in severe diarrhea in a child of this age
    B. Describe the medical problem to the boy in simple, easy-to-understand language
    C. Explain to the boy's mother the nature of the problem and the important features of the pathogen involved
    D. Instruct the boy's mother to give the boy fluids and schedule a follow-up appointment in 1 week
    E. Provide the boy's mother with a prescription for the appropriate antibiotic
    F. Refer the boy to an infectious disease specialist

12. A 56-year-old executive complains to his physician that he has had trouble sleeping for several months. His insomnia has become disruptive to both his professional and personal life. He mentions that a friend of his was given a prescription for benzodiazapines by his physician for a similar problem, and asks you to give him the same medication to "make this go away." The physician's best response would be to

    A. assess his current level of alcohol intake
    B. ask him about any recent stressors in his life
    C. inquire about the specifics of the insomnia
    D. give him some free samples of the medication he requests so he can try it out
    E. provide him with the prescription he requests
    F. instruct him to get more physical exercise
    G. refer him to a local psychiatrist for evaluation and counseling

13. A 24-year-old woman is scheduled for delivery by Cesarean section after her unborn child is determined to be wedged in a breech position. Prior to the surgery, the woman asks the physician to pray with her, and to carry a "charm," a dried animal tongue, with him as he performs the procedure. The physician is not religious and is taken aback by the request. He comes to you and asks your advice as to what he should do. Your best advice would be to tell him to

    A. advise the patient that her beliefs are not in keeping with modern medical practice
    B. go along with the patient's request by praying with her and carrying the charm
    C. politely explain to the patient that he does not share her religious beliefs
    D. pray with her and tell her he will carry the charm, but leave it outside the operating theater for sanitary reasons
    E. schedule an appointment for the patient with the appropriate hospital chaplain
    F. stand in the room as she prays, but decline to carry the charm
    G. suggest to the patient that she might be more comfortable with another physician performing the procedure

Answers and Explanations

1. **Answer: A.** Alcohol abuse suppresses REM sleep. REM sleep increases for major depression. L-tryptophan decreases sleep latency. Lithium carbonate should increase REM as it allows the manic patient to get more sleep. Anxiety by itself has no demonstrated effect on REM.

2. **Answer: C.** Although often given to help patients to go to sleep, paradoxically, one of the side effects of sedative hypnotic medication is insomnia with long-term use.

3. **Answer: B.** By age 2 to 3 years, about 25% of the child's sleep time is spent in REM sleep. This sleep is characterized by several sleep periods totaling about 11 (less than 15) hours of sleep in each 24-hour period. Stage 4 sleep is present at birth. The 90-minute sleep cycle is achieved only during the teenage years.

4. **Answer: E.** Stage 2 sleep is characterized by sleep spindles and K-complexes. Delta waves go with stages 3 and 4. Theta waves are stage 1. Sawtooth waves appear in REM.

5. **Answer: B.** Human growth hormone and serotonin levels rise during the first 3 hours of sleep.

6. **Answer: E.** The increased cerebral temperature that results from exercise is associated with increased delta sleep.

7. **Answer: G.** These symptoms suggest sleep apnea. The age of the patient and the loud snoring indicate obstructive apnea.

8. **Answer: G.** Take time to find out about the patient.

9. **Answer: G.** Do not give a prescription before evaluating the patient. If your office hours are an impediment for the patient, see him outside of normal office hours.

10. **Answer: B.** Faced with an irate patient, the rule is to express empathy, then give control.

11. **Answer: C.** Before discussing treatment, be sure that the patient understands the problem. Discuss the disease before discussing treatment.

12. **Answer: C.** Get the details about the patient's condition before proceeding to treatment. Of course you will not give medication just because the patient asks for it. You must be sure that it is needed.

13. **Answer: B.** Participating in the patient's religion is associated with better patient outcomes.

11 Diagnostic and Statistical Manual (DSM-5)

Learning Objectives

- ❑ Demonstrate understanding of applying child-development principles
- ❑ List the major categories of psychiatric disease as defined by DSM-5
- ❑ Give examples of disorders within each category, including their epidemiology, course, and treatment
- ❑ Answer questions about personality disorders

DISORDERS USUALLY DIAGNOSED IN CHILDHOOD

Intellectual Disability

The most common known cause of intellectual disability is **fetal alcohol syndrome** (FAS), while the most common genetic causes are **Down** and **fragile-X syndromes**.

Table 11-1. Intellectual Disability

Level	IQ	Functioning
Mild	70–50	Self-supporting with some guidance; 85% of intellectually disabled; male:female ratio 2: 1; usually diagnosed first year in school
Moderate	49–35	Benefits from vocational training, but needs supervision; sheltered workshops
Severe	34–20	Vocational training not helpful, can learn to communicate, basic self-care habits
Profound	<20	Needs highly structured environment, constant nursing care, and supervision

Autism Spectrum Disorders

Formerly called *pervasive development* disorders, these occur in 1 of every 150 births and are usually diagnosed age<3. Male:female ratio is 4:1. Clinical signs include:

- Problems with reciprocal social interaction, decreased repetoire of activities and interests
- Abnormal or delayed language development, impairment in verbal and nonverbal communication
- No separation anxiety
- Oblivious to external world
- Fails to assume anticipatory posture, shrinks from touch
- Pronoun reversal
- Preference for inanimate objects
- Stereotyped behavior and interests

With autism spectrum disorders, there is a link to chromosomes #15 and #11. Monozygotic concordance is greater than dizygotic concordance. IQ is <70 in 80% of those affected. Potential causes include association with prenatal/perinatal injury, e.g., rubella in first trimester and a mother who had asthma, allergies, or psoriasis while pregnant (2x more likely).

Differential diagnosis: Rett's: g > b, hand-wringing, microcephaly

In autism spectrum disorder without language impairment (formerly *Asperger's*), language is normal, IQ is normal, and there is a higher level of functioning.

Treatment: behavioral techniques (shaping) and risperidone (reduces agitation/aggression)

Note

Definitions

- **Anhedonia:** can't experience or even imagine any pleasant emotion
- **Clang associations:** illogical connections by rhythm or puns
- **Delusions:** false beliefs not shared by culture
- **Echolalia:** repeating in answer many of same words as in question
- **Echopraxia:** imitations of movements or gestures
- **Flight of ideas:** topics strung together
- **Hallucinations:** sensory impression, no stimuli
- **Illusions:** misperception of real stimuli
- **Loose associations:** jump from one topic to the next
- **Mannerisms,** e.g., grimacing
- **Mutism:** no speech
- **Neologisms:** new expressions
- **Perseveration:** responding to all questions the same way
- **Poverty of speech:** sparse and slow speech
- **Pressured speech:** abundant and accelerated speech
- **Verbigeration:** senseless repetition of same words or phrases

Attention Deficit Hyperactivity Disorder

Attention deficit hyperactivity disorder (ADHD) is marked by problems with inattention, impulsivity, and hyperactivity. Male-to-female ratio is 10:1. It is associated with low dopamine levels.

Treatment: methylphenidate, dextroamphetamine, atomoxetine

SCHIZOPHRENIA

The criteria for schizophrenia include bizarre delusions, auditory hallucinations (in 75%), blunted affect, loose associations, deficiency in reality testing, distorted perception, impaired functioning overall, and disturbance in behavior and form and content of language and thought for >6 months duration.

Note that if symptoms <6 months, it is **schizophreniform disorder**. If symptoms >1 day and <30 days, it is **brief psychotic disorder**.

Age of onset is age 15–24 (males) and 25–34 (females). Prevalence is 1% of the population cross-culturally; however, it is less chronic and less severe in developing countries than in developed countries. There is a downward drift to low SES.

- Around half of patients attempt suicide and 10% succeed
- Over 50% of schizophrenics do not live with their families but are not institutionalized

Genetic contribution:

- Rates for monozygotic twins reared apart = rates for MZ twins raised together (47%)
- Dizygotic concordance: 13%
- If 2 schizophrenic parents: 40% incidence
- If 1 parent or 1 sibling: 12%
- **Heritability index:** $\frac{MZ-DZ}{100-DZ}$ = proportion of conditions due to genetic factors
- Risk in biologic relatives 10x general population (i.e., 10%)

Clinical Presentation

DSM-5 does not include subtypes of schizophrenia. Rather, current severity is documented from 0 (low) to 4 (high) for the following 5 symptoms:

- Delusions
- Hallucinations
- Disorganized speech
- Abnormal psychomotor activity
- Negative symptoms

Paranoid symptoms include delusions of persecution or grandeur, often accompanied by hallucinations (voices).

Catatonic symptoms include **complete stupor** or pronounced decrease in spontaneous movements; possible muteness; frequent negativism, echopraxia, automatic obedience; rigidity of posture (can stand or sit in awkward position for long period of time). **Alternatively**, symptoms can include **excitedness** with evidence of extreme motor agitation:

- Incoherence with possible violence or destruction
- In their excitedness, self-harm or collapse into exhaustion
- Repetitious, stereotyped behaviors

It is important to understand the following clinical terms:

- **Positive symptoms** (type I): **what schizophrenic persons have that nonaffected individuals do not**, e.g., delusions, hallucinations, bizarre behavior; these are associated with **dopamine receptors**
- **Negative symptoms** (type II): **what nonaffected individuals have that schizophrenics do not**, e.g., flat affect, motor retardation, apathy, mutism; these are associated with **muscarinic receptors**

The following are **predictors for good prognosis** of schizophrenia:

- Paranoid symptoms
- Late onset (female)
- Quick onset
- Positive symptoms
- No family history of schizophrenia
- Family history of mood disorder
- Absence of structural brain abnormalities

Neurochemical Issues

The **dopamine hypothesis** is based on the effectiveness of neuroleptic medications in ameliorating the symptoms of schizophrenia; the correlation of clinical efficacy with drug potency in dopamine receptor antagonists; findings of increased dopamine receptor sensitivity in postmortem studies; and PET scan studies of schizophrenic patients compared with controls.

Role of serotonin (5-HT): Genes involved in serotoninergic neurotransmission are implicated in the pathogenesis of schizophrenia. LSD affects serotonin and can produce a psychotic-like state. Newer antipsychotics (e.g., clozapine) have high affinity for serotonin receptors. Serotonin rises when dopamine falls in some areas of the brain.

Role of glutamate: Major neurotransmitter in pathways key to schizophrenic symptoms. *N*-methyl-D-aspartate (NMDA) receptors; regulates brain development and controls apoptosis. Phencyclidine and ketamine block the NMDA channel: these can create positive and negative psychotic symptoms identical to schizophrenia. Drugs which indirectly enhance NMDA receptor function can reduce negative symptoms and improve cognitive function. 2-(aminomethyl) phenylacetic acid (AMPA) receptors:

- Abnormally sparse in temporal lobes of schizophrenics
- Ampakines selectively enhance transmission and improve memory in patients

Attention and Information Processing Deficits

There are 2 major processing deficits seen in schizophrenic patients:

- **Smooth pursuit eye movement (SPEM) impairment**
  - While unaffected individuals are able to follow a slow-moving target without error, up to 80% of schizophrenic patients and 50% of their relatives show saccadic eye movement and deficits at this tracking task.
- **Prefrontal cortical (PFC) impairment**
  - While unaffected individuals who are faced with a cognitive task will have increased activity in the prefrontal cortex, schizophrenic patients show decreased physiologic activity when faced with these tasks.
  - Impaired performance is seen on Wisconsin Card Sort (WCST), a test sensitive to prefrontal dysfunction.

- Clinical profile has similarities with patients with frontal lobe injury (e.g., cognitive inflexibility, problem-solving difficulties, and apathy).

Structural and Anatomic Abnormalities in the Brain

Cortical abnormalities include larger ventricle size and ventricular brain ratios (VBRs), cortical atrophy, smaller frontal lobes, atrophy of temporal lobes, and an association with specific clinical and cognitive correlates e.g., deficit symptoms, cognitive impairment, and poor outcome:

- Correlation between ventricle size, type, and prognosis of illness
- More dilation with negative symptoms
- However, dilated ventricles also reported among patients having unipolar, bipolar, and schizoaffective disorders (sensitive, but not specific indicator)

Subtle anomalies in limbic structures (the limbic system is seen as the **site of the primary pathology for schizophrenia**);

- Changes in hippocampus, parahippocampal gyrus, entorhinal cortex, amygdala, cingulate gyrus
- Smaller volume of left hippocampus and amygdala
- Also found in high-risk, nonsymptomatic patients

Treatment: antipsychotic medications reduce acute (positive) symptoms in 75% of patients with schizophrenia, versus 25% with placebo. Relapse rates are about 40% in 2 years if on medication and 80% in 2 years if off medication. The prognosis is mixed: 33% of patients lead normal lives, 33% experience symptoms but function in society, and 33% require frequent hospitalization.

DEPRESSIVE DISORDERS AND BIPOLAR AND RELATED DISORDERS (MOOD DISORDERS)

Depression and elation are normal human emotions. They are disordered when they get too long-term or too extreme.

Table 11-2. Mood Disorders

	Mild	Severe
Stable	Persistent Depressive Disorder	Major depression
Alternating	Cyclothymia	Bipolar (manic-depression)

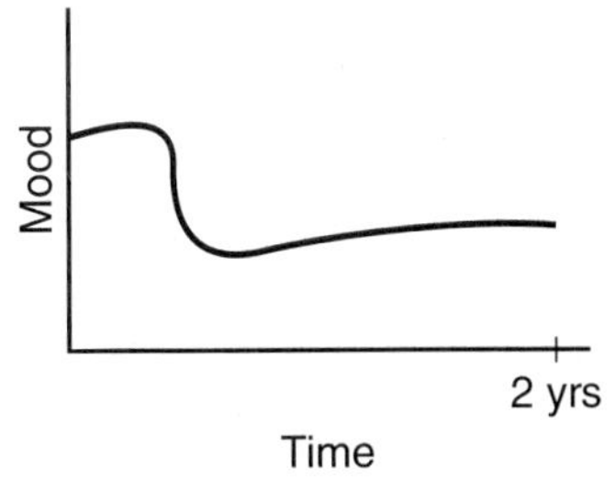

Subtypes

Persistent depressive disorder

- Chronic (at least 2 years); patient is functional but at suboptimal level
- Depressed mood on most days for >2 years
- Not severe enough for hospitalization
- Lifetime prevalence 5%

Cyclothymia

- >2 years
- Alternating states between depressed moods and hypomania

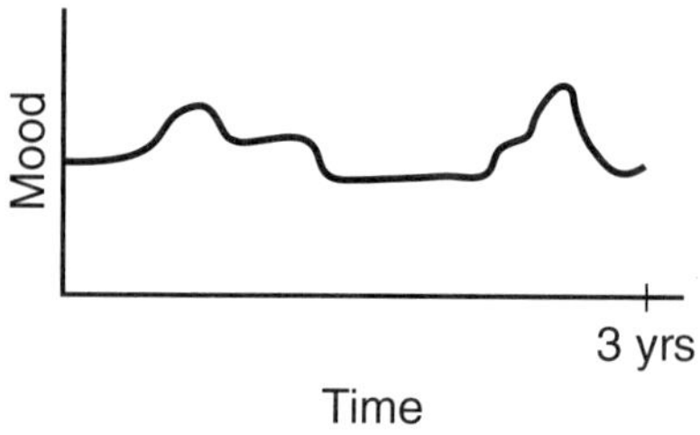

Depression with seasonal pattern (seasonal affective disorder)

- Depressive symptoms during months with short or long days
- May be related to abnormal melatonin metabolism
- Treat with bright light therapy (not melatonin tablets)

Major depressive disorder

- Symptoms for at least 2 weeks
- Must represent a change from previous functioning
- May be associated with anhedonia, lack of motivation, feelings of worthlessness, decreased concentration, weight loss or gain, depressed mood, recurrent thoughts, insomnia or hypersomnia, psychomotor agitation or retardation, somatic complains, delusions or hallucinations (if mood congruent), and loss of sex drive
- Suicide: 60% of depressed patients have suicidal ideation and 15% die by suicide
- Decrease in most hormones
- Neurochemical changes include decrease in norepinephrine, seotonin, dopamine (and all related metabolites)
- Sleep correlates:
  - Increased REM in first half of sleep
  - Decreased REM latency
  - Increased REM time overall
  - Decreased stage 4 sleep
  - Early morning waking

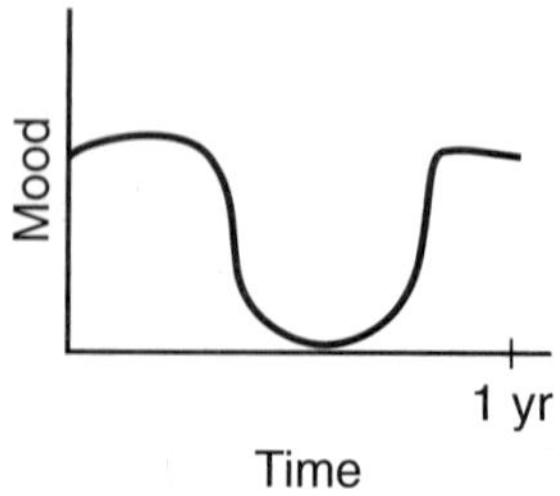

Bipolar disorder

- Symptoms of major depression **plus** symptoms of mania: a period of abnormal and persistent elevated, expansive, or irritable mood; i.e., alternates between depression and mania
- Subtypes are **bipolar I (mania and major depression)** and **bipolar II (major depression plus hypomanic episodes)**

- Manic symptoms include increased self-esteem or grandiosity, low frustration tolerance, decreased need for sleep, flight of ideas, excessive involvement in activities, weight loss and anorexia, erratic and uninhibited behavior, and increased libido
- Neurochemical changes include increased norepinephrine and increased serotonin
- Markedly decreased sleep time; multiple awakenings
- Most genetic of all psychiatric disorders

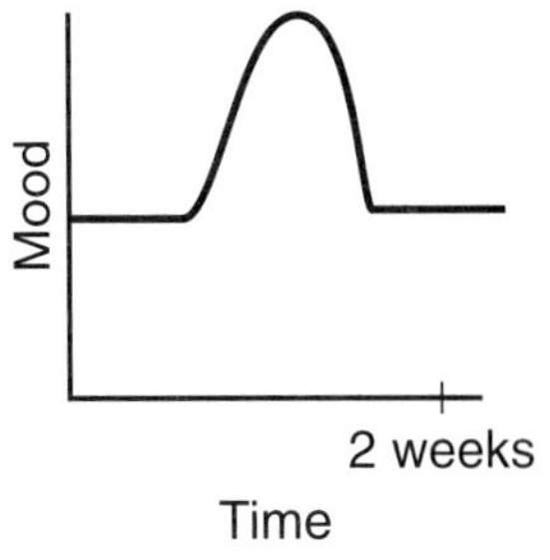

Table 11-3. Epidemiology of Mood Disorders

	Depression	Bipolar
Point prevalence	Men: 2–3%, women: 5–9%	Men and women <1%
Gender differences	Women 2× men (stress of childbirth, hormonal effects, abused as children)	Rates are effectively equal
Lifetime prevalence	Men 10%, women 20%	Men and women 1%
Onset	Mean age 40	Mean age 30
SES	Low SES more likely	Higher SES more likely
Relationships	More prevalent among those with no close relationships, separation, divorce	More prevalent among single and divorced (causal?)
Family history	Higher risk if parents depressed or alcoholic; increased risk if parental loss age <11	Higher risk if parent has bipolar

EATING DISORDERS

Bulimia nervosa is the compulsive, rapid ingestion of food followed by compensatory behavior such as self-induced vomiting, use of laxatives, or exercise. In other words, binge and purge. It is seen in ~4% females and 0.5% males; 5–10% of women experience it at some point during their lives. It is often associated with girls who previously were obese.

If there is no compensatory behavior, the diagnosis is **binge-eating disorder**, not bulimia.

Clinical signs of bulimia include scars on back of hands, esophageal tears, enlarged parotid gland, and minimal public eating. Personality is outgoing and impulsive. Low baseline serotonin concentrations are often seen (repeated binges raise serotonin). Around 35% have a drug or alcohol problem.

Treatment: SSRIs, insight, and group therapy

Anorexia nervosa is characterized by self-imposed dietary limitations, significant weight loss (15–20% below ideal body weight); i.e., self-starvation (BMI <17.5). There is a fear of gaining weight; patient "feels fat" even when she is very thin (body image disturbance). The appearance of lanugo (baby-fine hair) is characteristic. It is seen in 0.5% of the population (95% are female); 2% of adolescent females; primarily ages 10–30 (far majority are age 13–20), and is uncommon in women age >40. Mortality is 5–18%.

Predisposing factors are family dynamics linked to relationship with father/harsh mother and a mother with history (50% of susceptibility is inherited). Around 50% of anorexics also binge and purge.

Treatment: patients are usually resistant to treatment (denial of illness); full treatment is to stabilize weight, then do family and individual therapy. Pharmacologic treatment may include antidepressants (to cause weight gain).

Table 11-4. Eating Disorders

	Anorexia Nervosa	Bulimia Nervosa
Gender	W > M	W > M
Age	Mid-teenage years	Late adolescence/early adulthood
SES	Not specific to high	Not specific to high
Weight	>15% below ideal body weight	Varies, usually nl. or >nl.
Neurotransmitters	Serotonin/norepinephrine?	Serotonin/norepinephrine?
Binge/purge	Yes	Yes
Laxative/diuretics	Yes	Yes
Sexual adjustment	Poor	Good
Medical complications	• Amenorrhea • Lanugo • High mortality • Dental cavities • Electrolyte imbalances	• Electrolyte imbalances • Dental cavities • Callous on hands/fingers • Enlarged parotid and salivary glands • Cardiac abnormalities

ANXIETY DISORDERS

Anxiety disorders are the most common psychiatric disorders in women of all ages. In men, substance-related disorders are the most common.

With **generalized anxiety disorder**, symptoms are exhibited more days than not over a period of 6 months (patient worries about things he does not need to worry about). Symptoms include motor tension (fidgety, jumpy), autonomic hyperactivity (heart pounding, sweating, chest pains), hyperventilation, apprehension (fear, worry, rumination), difficulty concentrating, vigilance and scanning (impatient, hyperactive, distracted), fatigue, and sleep disturbances such as insomnia. Treatment: SSRI or buspirone.

Panic disorder (1.5% of population with 4% lifetime prevalence) is defined as 3 anxiety attacks in a 3-week period (and the patient worries about having even more). There is no clear circumscribed stimulus; it is a phobic-level reaction without a phobic object. Onset of symptoms is abrupt and peaks within 10 minutes: great apprehension/fear, palpitations, trembling, sweating, fear of dying or going crazy, hyperventilation, "air hunger," and a sense of unreality.

- Affects young women
- 2x more common in those with allergies
- Premenstrual period: heightened vulnerability
- Can induce panic attacks by hyperventilation, carbon dioxide, yohimbine, sodium lactate, epinephrine (panicogens)

Treatment: alprazolam, clonazepam, lorazepam; SSRIs, carbon dioxide (for hyperventilation) (relapse is common so keep on medication for 6–12 months)

Phobias

Phobias are seen in 4% of men and 9% of women. Public speaking is the #1 phobia.

Specific phobias include fear of a specific object, e.g., spiders or snakes. Anxiety is experience in when faced with the identifiable object; phobic object is thus avoided. The fear must be persistent and disabling. Treat with behavior modification (systematic desensitization, exposure, flooding).

Social anxiety disorder (1% of population) includes fear of being embarrassed or humiliated. It leads to dysfunctional circumspect behavior, e.g., an inability to urinate in public washrooms, go to restaurants, and speak in public. Social anxiety disorder may accompany avoidant personality disorder. Treat with SSRI or beta blocker (atenolol, propranolol) for discrete performance anxiety such as stage fright.

OBSESSIVE–COMPULSIVE DISORDER AND RELATED DISORDERS

In **obsessive-compulsive disorder** (1.5% of population 3% lifetime prevalence), there is **obsession** (thoughts which are repetitive, intrusive, and senseless) and **compulsion** (act which controls the thought and is time-consuming). Common defenses are undoing, reaction formation.

- 50% of patients remain unmarried
- Males = females
- 70% experience major depression over lifetime

There is increased frontal lobe metabolism and increased activity in the caudate nucleus. Treatment is SSRIs.

Hoarding disorder is characterized by persistent difficulty with parting of one's possessions, regardless of their value. This typically leads to changes in functioning. Treatment is SSRIs.

In **body dysmorphic disorder**, the patient believes a body part is abnormal, misshapen, or defective; sees self as ugly or horrific when normal in appearance. Preoccupation disrupts day-to-day life. It is not accounted for by other disorders (e.g., anorexia nervosa). Patient may seek multiple plastic surgeries or other extreme interventions.

TRAUMA AND STRESS-RELATED DISORDERS

Manifestations of trauma or a stress-related disorder include re-experiencing of the event as a recurrent dream or recollection (flashbacks), avoidance of associated stimuli, diminished responsiveness to the external world, sleep disruption or excess, irritability, loss of control, impulsivity, headaches, and inability to concentrate.

Symptoms must be exhibited for >1 month; if less, it should be diagnosed as acute stress disorder.

- Follows a psychologically stressful event outside the range of normal human experience; most commonly, serious threat to life, family, children, home, or community
- Common reaction to rape war, earthquakes, etc.
- Often long latency period, e.g., abused as child, manifest symptoms as an adult
- Quicker onset correlates with better prognosis
- Increased vulnerability if prior emotional variability; excessive autonomic reactions is a predictor of occurrence
- Adults recover more quickly; very young and very old have harder time coping
- Prevalence: 0.5% in men, 1.2% in women
- Sleep changes: increase in REM latency; decrease in amount of REM and Stage 4 sleep
- Increased, sustained activity in amygdala
- Increased levels of norepinephrine and epinephrine
- Decreased cortisol levels
- Co-occurrence with other psychiatric disorders common

Treatment: group therapy to facilitate working through normal reactions blocked by disorder. SSRIs can improve patients' functional level.

SOMATIC SYMPTOM DISORDERS, FACTITIOUS DISORDER, AND MALINGERING

Somatic Symptom Disorders

Somatic symptom disorder is defined as ≥1 somatic symptoms distressing enough to cause changes in level of functioning, as well as excessive and disproportionate thoughts, feelings, and behavior regarding those symptoms.

- Must be present >6 months
- Onset age <30
- Symptoms can occur over a period of years
- Females > males (20:1)

Conversion disorder (functional neurological symptom disorders) involves a stressor followed by ≥1 symptoms. It usually involves the skeletal, muscular, sensory, or peripheral nonautonomic system, e.g., paralysis of hand or loss of sight. Look for *la belle indifference.*

In **illness anxiety disorder**, there is a preoccupation with illness (or fear of illness) when none is present; the preoccupation persists in spite of reassurance. It is an unrealistic interpretation of physical symptoms/signs as being abnormal. Must be present >6 months.

In **somatic symptom disorder with predominant pain**, there is no cause found for severe, prolonged pain. The pain disrupts one's day-to-day life. Rule out depression and look for secondary gain.

Table 11-5. Somatic Symptom Disorders vs. Factitious Disorders and Malingering

	Somatic Symptom	Factitious	Malingering
Symptom production	Unconscious	Intentional	Intentional
Motivation	Unconscious	Unconscious	Intentional

Factitious Disorder

In factitious disorder, symptom production is both conscious and some unconscious. There is intentional illness production and unconscious motivation (therefore, a compulsion). Patients are aware of manufacturing their symptoms but unaware of why they go to such lengths. There is both primary and secondary gain.

Types:

- Imposed on self.
- Imposed on others (inducing symptoms in others e.g., a mother producing symptoms in her child)

Factitious disorders require treatment; foster the relationship and look for a motive.

Malingering

Everything is conscious, with intentional symptom production for gain. Conscious motivation. Symptoms are purely for secondary gain, e.g., to avoid a court date, military induction, or school.

ADJUSTMENT DISORDER

Adjustment disorder is a residual category, ie, use this *only* if no other diagnosis applies. Criteria are as follows:

- Presence of an identifiable stressor and symptoms within 3 months of onset
- Symptoms that last <6 months after the end of stressor
- Symptoms are clinically significant, with significant social, occupational, and/or academic impairment
- Cannot be a grief response and cannot meet criteria for another disorder

DISSOCIATIVE DISORDERS

Dissociative disorders use the defense mechanism of dissociation where a group of activities/thoughts is split off from the main part of consciousness. It is typically due to traumatic events.

Fugue involves sudden unexpected travel, an inability to recall one's past, or confusion of identity.

Subtypes (fugue state may appear with all subtypes):

- **Amnesia**: inability to recall important personal information
- **Dissociative identity disorder** (multiple personality): presence of two or more distinct identities; will have lapses in memory
- **Depersonalization disorder**: recurrent experiences of being detached from or outside of one's body—"out of body experiences"; reality testing stays intact; causes significant impairment

PERSONALITY DISORDERS

Personality disorders are maladaptive patterns of behavior; behaviors are ego-syntonic. General characteristics include inflexibility, inability to adapt; one way of responding. These disorders are lifelong and affect all areas of life.

Cluster A: Odd or Eccentric

This type has a higher prevalence in males and in biologic relatives of schizophrenics.

Paranoid

Long-standing suspiciousness or mistrust of others: a base line of mistrust. Preoccupied with issues of trust; reluctant to confide in others. Reads hidden meaning into comments or events. Carries grudges.

- Paranoid schizophrenic has hallucinations and formal thought disorders; paranoid personality disorder does not
- Delusional disorder, paranoid type has fixed, focal delusions; paranoid personality disorder does not

Schizoid

Lifelong pattern of social withdrawal, and they like it that way. Seen by others as eccentric, isolated, withdrawn. Restricted emotional expression.

Schizotypal

Very odd, strange, weird. Magical thinking (including ESP and telepathy), ideas of reference, illusions. Social anxiety (paranoid); suspiciousness; lack of close friends. Incongruous affect; odd speech; social isolation. May have short-lived psychotic episodes.

Cluster B: Dramatic and Emotional

Histrionic

Colorful, dramatic, extroverted, with inability to maintain long-lasting relationships. Attention-seeking, constantly wanting the spotlight; seductive behavior.

Narcissistic

Grandiose sense of self-importance. Preoccupation with fantasies of unlimited wealth, power, love. Demands constant attention; fragile self-esteem, prone to depression. Criticism met with indifference or rage. Genuine surprise and anger when others don't do as they want. Can be charismatic.

Borderline

Females > males 2:1. Very unstable affect, behavior, self-image; in constant state of crisis, chaos. Self-detrimental impulsivity: promiscuity, gambling, overeating, substance-related disorders. Unstable but intense interpersonal relationships: very dependent and hostile, love/hate.

- Great problems with being alone
- Self-injurious behavior
- History of sexual abuse
- Common defenses: splitting, passive–aggressive
- Particularly incapable of tolerating anxiety
- Often coupled with mood disorder
- 5% commit suicide

Antisocial

Affects 3% males, 1% females. Continual criminal acts. Inability to conform to social norms: truancy, delinquency, theft, running away. Can't hold job, no enduring attachments, reckless, aggressive. Onset age <15; if age <18, diagnose as conduct disorder.

Cluster C: Anxious and Fearful

These behaviors are associated with fear and anxiety.

Avoidant

Extreme sensitivity to rejection; sees self as socially inept. Excessive shyness, high anxiety levels. Social isolation, but an intense, internal desire for affection and acceptance. Wants the world to change, to be nicer, more accepting. Tends to stay in same job, same life situation, same relationships.

Obsessive–compulsive

Orderliness, inflexible, perfectionist; more common in males, firstborn, harsh discipline upbringing. Loves lists, rules, order. Unable to discard worn-out objects. Doesn't want change; excessively stubborn; lacks sense of humor. Wants to keep routine. Differentiate from obsessive–compulsive anxiety disorder. The anxiety disorder has obsessions and compulsions that are focal and acquired. Personality disorders are lifelong and pervasive.

Dependent

Gets others to assume responsibility; subordinates own needs to others. Can't express disagreement. Great fear of having to care for self. May be linked to abusive spouse.

Table 11-6. Personality Disorders

	Definition	Epidemiology	Associated Defenses
Paranoid	Attributes involvement motives to others, suspicious	Men > women; increased incidence in families with schizophrenia	Projection
Schizoid	Isolated lifestyle, has no longing for others, "loner"	Men > women; increased incidence in families with schizophrenia	
Schizotypal	Weird, eccentric behavior, thought, speech	Prevalence 3%; men > women	
Histrionic	Excessive emotion and attention seeking	Women > men; underdiagnosed in men	
Narcissistic	Grandiose, overconcerned with issues of self-esteem	Common	
Borderline	Instability of mood, selfimage, and relationships	Women > men; increased mood disorders in families	Splitting
Antisocial	Does not recognize the rights of others	Prevalence: 3% men; 1% women	Superego lacunae
Avoidant	Shy or timid, fears rejection	Common; possible deforming illness	
Dependent	Dependent, submissive	Common; women > men	
Obssessive-compulsive	Perfectionistic and inflexible, orderly, rigid	Men > women; increased concordance in identical twins	Undoing; reaction formation

Review Questions

1. A 6-year-old boy was referred by his first grade teacher for evaluation after she noticed that he had trouble keeping up with the other children in his class. After psychologic testing and an evaluation interview, the boy's IQ is assessed at 62. Based on this information, when he is an adult the boy most likely will

   A. find work in a sheltered workshop setting
   B. have difficulty with basic reading and math skills
   C. lead a normal life with no special support required
   D. require custodial care
   E. need guidance for important life decisions

2. A 45-year-old woman presents to her primary care physician complaining of fatigue and headaches. Over the past month, she reports that she has had trouble sleeping, difficulty concentrating, and episodes of crying for no reason. In addition, she says that she feels sad and worthless. The neurologic pathway most likely implicated as the source of these symptoms is the

   A. meso-limbic-cortico pathway
   B. locus ceruleus pathway
   C. nigrostriatal pathway
   D. nucleus accumbens pathway
   E. glycolytic pathway

3. A 42-year-old woman has always been extremely neat and conscientious, skills she makes good use of as the executive secretary to the president of a large corporation. Something of a perfectionist, she often stays long after normal working hours to check on the punctuation and spelling of letters that she prepared during the day. Although her work is impeccable, she has few close relationships with others. Her boss referred her for counseling after she repeatedly got into fights with her coworkers. "They just don't take the job to heart," she says disapprovingly about them. "All they seem to want to do is joke around all day." The most likely preliminary diagnosis for this patient is

   A. obsessive–compulsive personality disorder
   B. paranoid personality disorder
   C. schizoid personality disorder
   D. hysterical personality disorder
   E. antisocial personality disorder
   F. narcissistic personality disorder
   G. borderline personality disorder
   H. dependent personality disorder
   I. avoidant personality disorder
   J. schizotypal personality disorder

4. A 22-year-old male patient refuses to provide answers to standard questions during an initial history and physical exam, including address and telephone number. When asked the reason for the refusal, he says he doesn't see why the physician needs such irrelevant information and eyes the physician suspiciously. When pressed further, he asks angrily, "Look, are you going to treat me or do I have to get my lawyer?" This behavior is most consistent with a diagnosis of

   A. obsessive–compulsive personality disorder
   B. paranoid personality disorder
   C. schizoid personality disorder
   D. hysterical personality disorder
   E. antisocial personality disorder
   F. narcissistic personality disorder
   G. borderline personality disorder
   H. dependent personality disorder
   I. avoidant personality disorder
   J. schizotypal personality disorder

5. A patient's past medical history indicates numerous admissions to a local public hospital, mostly during the winter months. On each occasion, he has been brought to the hospital after passing out in a public location. His appearance is disheveled and his clothes are torn. He complains that the cold makes him dizzy and asks the physician, with tears in his eyes, to "please help him get better." Neurologic examination is unable to uncover any underlying cause for his reported symptoms. The most likely preliminary diagnosis for this patient would be

   A. dysthymia
   B. somatic symptom disorder
   C. delusional disorder
   D. factitious disorder
   E. malingering

6. A man awakens to find a bright sunny day. As he dresses, he makes sure to put on a yellow shirt to ensure that it will stay sunny all day. This behavior can best be described as

   A. delusion
   B. hallucination
   C. idea of reference
   D. magical thinking
   E. illusion

7. Glenn has been a model patient on the ward for more than 2 years. He is never in any trouble. Whatever he is told to do he does. He sits quietly for hours, rarely talking, and hardly moving, except to ape the movements of those who pass by him. The most likely diagnosis for Glenn is

   A. schizophreniform disorder
   B. schizoid personality disorder
   C. brief psychotic disorder
   D. schizotypal personality disorder
   E. schizophrenia, catatonic specifier

8. According to twin studies, the strongest evidence of a genetic cause is for

   A. schizophrenia
   B. bipolar disorder
   C. unipolar depression
   D. antisocial personality disorder
   E. alcoholism

9. A patient suffering from paranoid schizophrenia has been on his medication for a full year. During this time, his positive symptoms have abated and he shows no signs of relapse. If he continues to be adherent with his medication, his chance of relapse over the coming years is most likely to be

   A. 80%
   B. 50%
   C. 40%
   D. 30%
   E. 10%

10. A 22-year-old intellectually disabled male lives on his own but works in a sheltered workshop setting. He has an active social life and is well liked by his peers. He meets weekly with a counselor who helps him handle his money and provides advice about some life decisions. Based on this information, this man will most likely be considered as having what level of intellectual disability?

    A. Below average
    B. Mild
    C. Moderate
    D. Severe
    E. Profound

11. A 38-year-old woman is brought by her husband to see her primary care physician. The husband reports that she is getting hard to live with. Physical exam reveals rapid heartbeat and profuse sweating. In conversation, the woman has a hard time focusing and gets up from her chair repeatedly. After some time, she reports that she is tired and has had difficulty sleeping for "what seems like a year, now." She attributes this difficulty sleeping to her tendency to worry about her children and confides that she checks on them 10 to 20 times a night. When questioned about friends, she states that she just doesn't see them much any more. Based on this preliminary information, the most likely diagnosis for this woman would be

    A. agoraphobia
    B. generalized anxiety disorder
    C. social anxiety disorder
    D. obsessive–compulsive disorder
    E. panic disorder

12. A 42-year-old man who makes his living as a computer programmer and works out of his own home is referred by his employer for evaluation. He is reluctant to venture out to meet with other people, and rarely has people in to visit. When selected for a company-wide award, he refuses to have his picture taken for the company newsletter. During an assessment interview, he averts his face and asks the examiner to "stop looking at me." Although he is average in appearance, he is convinced that his face is ugly and misshapen and says that he stays away from people so they "won't have to look at me." The most likely diagnosis for this man would be

    A. agoraphobia
    B. body dysmorphic disorder
    C. factitious disorder
    D. obsessive–compulsive disorder
    E. social anxiety disorder
    F. somatic symptom disorder

13. A young woman of unknown age is brought by the police to the local emergency department for evaluation after they found her wandering in a local park. The woman carries no purse and no identification. Physical exam shows no abnormalities. When questioned, the woman is pleasant and attentive, making eye contact and answering each question as it is asked. She is unable to state her name or any details about her life, except that the name Phoenix seems familiar, although she is not sure why. The police in Phoenix, Arizona, are contacted and find a missing persons report matching the patient's description. Based on this information, the most likely diagnosis for this patient is

    A. adjustment disorder
    B. amnesia
    C. conversion disorder
    D. depersonalization disorder
    E. dissociative identity disorder
    F. factitious disorder
    G. dissociative amnesia with fugue

14. For 3 weeks following an automobile accident where she watched her child die, a 28-year-old woman reports difficulty sleeping, headaches, and an inability to concentrate. Her family reports that she suffers from nightmares and violent emotional outbursts when awake. Since the accident, she refuses to either drive or ride in a car. The symptoms presented here are most consistent with a diagnosis of

    A. adjustment disorder
    B. post-traumatic stress disorder
    C. acute stress disorder
    D. dysthymia
    E. major depression
    F. normal grief

15. A 28-year-old white male presents at a local clinic complaining of severe abdominal pain. He reports tenderness during palpation, dizziness, and difficulty concentrating. Review of the medical record shows that this is the fourth time in the past year that the patient has appeared for medical attention. On each previous occasion, no identifiable medical problem could be uncovered. When confronted with this history, the patient confesses that he manufactures his symptoms before coming to the clinic. He says that he knows this is wrong, but he cannot stop himself from doing this. Based on the information, the most likely diagnosis for this patient would be

    A. somatic symptom disorder
    B. conversion disorder
    C. illness anxiety disorder
    D. factitious disorder
    E. malingering

Answers and Explanations

1. **Answer: E.** The tested IQ suggests mild intellectual disability. These individuals live their own lives and make their own decisions, but often need assistance at some of life's important transitions points. Note that they are legally competent.

2. **Answer: B.** Starting in the retrolateral part of the pons, this is the major pathway for norepinepherine. Mesolimbic and nigrostriatal pathways are associated with dopamine and therefore, schizophrenia.

3. **Answer: A.** Focusing on details, loving routine, having a sense that there is only one right way to do things, lack of humor, and few close relationships suggests an obsessive–compulsive personality disorder.

4. **Answer: B.** General suspiciousness and mistrust suggests a paranoid personality disorder.

5. **Answer: E.** The timing during the winter months and the public venue for the passing out are all suggestive of the secondary gain of malingering.

6. **Answer: D.** The yellow shirt influences the sunny day. This is an example of magical thinking.

7. **Answer: E.** This is an example of schizophrenia with catatonic specifier.

8. **Answer: B.** The Heritability Index tells us that about 62% of bipolar disorder is due to inheritance. This is greater than schizophrenia (40%) and the other options.

9. **Answer: E.** If patients are compliant with medication and make it past the first year without relapse, the chance of relapse is a low 10%.

10. **Answer: C.** Moderate intellectual disability (IQ 49 to 35). He is able to take care of some of his own affairs, but needs weekly help with finances and works in a sheltered workshop.

11. **Answer: B.** The symptoms and timeframe are consistent with a diagnosis of generalized anxiety disorder. Although some features of other disorders are present, they do not match criteria.

12. **Answer: B.** The central issue is the negative appraisal of his own appearance. All other symptoms arise from this.

13. **Answer: G.** One of the dissociative disorders defined as sudden travel and inability to recall one's past or confusion about one's identity.

14. **Answer: C.** Avoidance of associated stimuli and nightmares after an identified traumatic event are the criteria for PTSD. But the timeframe, 3 weeks, makes acute stress disorder the better answer.

15. **Answer: D.** Factitious disorders are characterized by conscious symptom production and unconscious motivation. Somatic symptom disorder, conversion disorder, and illness anxiety disorder are all subtypes of somatic symptom disorders. Malingering is a conscious symptom production and there is clear, conscious secondary gain.

Organic Disorders 12

Learning Objectives

- ❑ Differentiate delirium, dementia, and psychosis
- ❑ Solve problems concerning hemispheric dominance and aphasias
- ❑ Solve problems concerning Tourette's disorder
- ❑ List the neuroanatomic areas of the brain and describe behaviors associated with each area
- ❑ List the major neurotransmitters, the areas and pathways of the nervous system they are associated with, and their correlation with observable behaviors

TOURETTE'S DISORDER

Tourette's disorder is characterized by multiple motor and vocal tics that occur many times every day or intermittently for >1 year. Tics can be simple (rapid, repetitive contractions) or complex (appear as more ritualistic and purposeful), and simple tics appear first.

- Prevalence is 0.5–1 per 1,000.
- Mean onset is age 7 (onset must be age <18).
- Male to female ratio is 3:1.
- Evidence of genetic transmission: ~50% concordance in monozygotic twins
- Associated with increased levels of dopamine
- Associated with ADHD and OCD
- Treatment: haloperidol, pimozide, or clonidine

DELIRIUM VERSUS NEUROCOGNITIVE DISORDER

Delirium: acute onset, impaired cognitive functioning, fluctuating and brief, reversible

Neurocognitive Disorder: loss of cognitive abilities, impaired social functioning, loss of memory, personality change; only 15% reversible; may be progressive or static

Table 12-1. Delirium versus Neurocognitive Disorder

	Delirium	Neurocognitive Disorder
History	Acute, identifiable date	Chronic, cannot be dated
Onset	Rapid	Insidious
Duration	Days to weeks	Months to years
Course	Fluctuating	Chronically progressive
Level of consciousness	Fluctuating	Normal
Orientation	Impaired periodically	Disorientationto time → place → person
Memory	Recent markedly impaired	Recent impaired then remote
Perception	Visual hallucinations	Hallucinations, sundowning
Sleep	Disrupted sleep-wake cycle	Less sleep disruption
Reversibility	Reversible	Most not reversible
Physiologic changes	Prominent	Minimal
Attention span	Very short	Not reduced

Neurocognitive Disorders

5% of population with neurocognitive disorders is older than 65, and 20% is older than 80; 15% of neurocognitive disorders are reversible.

Primary degenerative neurocognitive disorder of the Alzheimer type (DAT): DAT is most common; represents 65% of neurocognitive disorders in patients age >65. Prevalence increases with age, and women have a greater risk than men. Family history confers greater risk; there is less risk for higher educated. Linked to chromosomes 1 and 14 (mutations), 19 (apolipoprotein E), 21 (linked to Down syndrome).

Ten warning signs of Alzheimer disease:

- Memory loss that affects job skills
- Difficulty performing familiar tasks
- Problems with language
- Disorientation to time and place
- Poor judgment
- Problems with abstract thought
- Misplacing things
- Changes in mood or behavior
- Changes in personality
- Loss of initiative

Etiology is unknown. Theories include maternal age at birth, deficiency of brain choline, autoimmune disorders, viral etiology, and familial.

Gross pathology:

- Diffuse atrophy of the brain on CT or MRI
- Flattened cortical sulci
- Enlarged cerebral ventricles
- Deficient blood flow in parietal lobes correlated with cognitive decline
- Reduction in choline acetyl transferase
- Reduced metabolism in temporal and parietal lobes

Microscopic pathology:

- Accumulation of amyloid beta-peptides (protein fragment)
- Senile plaques
- Neurofibrillary tangles
- Granulovascular degeneration of the neurons
- Anatomic changes: to amygdala, hippocampus, cortex, basal forebrain

Treatment is supportive and symptomatic. Reduce environmental changes, hypertension, and LDL cholesterol levels. Treatment also includes donepezil hydrochloride, rivastigmine, galantamine, memantine.

Vascular neurocognitive disorder is decremental or patchy deterioration in cognitive functioning due to severe cerebrovascular disease. It is most prevalent between ages 60 and 70. Appears earlier than DAT. Men > women; hypertension is predisposing factor. 15% of all neurocognitive disorders in the elderly; lateralizing neurologic signs are often evident.

Vascular disease is present; affects small- and medium-sized cerebral vessels that infarct and produce parenchymal lesions over wide areas of the brain.

Treat underlying condition (hypertension, diabetes mellitus, hyperlipidemia); use general measures for neurocognitive disorder.

Table 12-2. Neurocognitive Disorder, Alzheimer Type versus Vascular Neurocognitive Disorder

Neurocognitive Disorder, Alzheimer Type	Vascular Neurocognitive Disorder
General deterioration	Patchy deterioration
More in women	More in men
Later onset	Earlier onset
Most common, 65% of neurocognitive disorders	Less common, 15% of neurocognitive disorders
Etiology unknown	Etiology features hypertension
Progressive onset	Quick onset
No lateral signs	Lateralizing neurologic signs

Frontal/temporal disease affects the frontal and temporal lobes. Very rare. Similar picture to neurocognitive disorder, Alzheimer type (DAT). Prominent frontal lobe symptoms (personality change). Reactive gliosis in frontal/temporal lobes; CT or MRI sometimes shows frontal lobe involvement but definitive diagnosis is only at autopsy.

Prion disease is a neurocognitive disorder caused by prion (no DNA or RNA). Rapidly progressive; generally onset between ages 40 and 50. Initially, vague somatic complaints and unspecified anxiety, followed by ataxia, choreoathetosis, and dysarthria. Fatal in 2 years (usually sooner). CT demonstrates atrophy in cortex/cerebellum. There is no treatment.

Huntington chorea: Autosomal dominant; defect in chromosome 4. Males = females. Basal ganglia and caudate atrophy; choreoathetoid movements, neurocognitive disorder, psychosis. Onset between ages 30 and 40. Progressive deterioration. Neurocognitive disorder, later with psychosis progressing to infantile state. Death in 15–20 years; suicide is common.

Parkinson's disease: Decreased dopamine in substantia nigra. Annual prevalence is 200 in 100,000. Symptoms:

- Bradykinesia
- Resting tremor
- Pill-rolling tremor
- Masklike facies
- Cogwheel rigidity
- Shuffling gait

About 40% to 80% develop a neurocognitive disorder.

Depression is common; treat with antidepressants or electroconvulsive therapy (ECT). Treatment is L-dopa or deprenyl.

Wilson disease: Defect in chromosome 13; ceruloplasmin deficiency. Abnormal copper metabolism; Kaiser-Fleischer rings.

Normal pressure hydrocephalus: Symptom triad of: neurocognitive disorder, urinary incontinence, gait apraxia (magnetic gait).

Increased ventricles on CT. Normal pressure on lumbar puncture.

Treat with shunt.

HIV-related neurocognitive disorder: Caused by chronic HIV encephalitis and myelitis. Two-thirds have insidious onset, one-third has florid onset. 70 to 95% of patients with AIDS have HIV-related neurocognitive disorder before death.

Clinically consists of the following:

- Cognitive symptoms: forgetfulness, loss of concentration, confusion
- Behavioral symptoms: apathy, withdrawal, dysphoric mood, organic psychosis
- Motor symptoms: loss of balance, leg weakness, poor handwriting

Average survival from onset to death is 4.2 months. Early signs of HIV-related neurocognitive disorder: dysphoric mood, apathy, social withdrawal. It is often misdiagnosed at first as depression. HIV levels in the spinal fluid are good predictors of onset.

HEMISPHERIC DOMINANCE

Left hemisphere: Dominant in language and calculation-type problem solving. Dominant in 97% of population, 60 to 70% in left-handed persons. Stroke damage to left is more likely to lead to depression; it is larger in size than the right side, and processes information faster.

Right hemisphere: Dominant in perception, artistic, and visual–spatial. Activated for intuition-type problem solving. Stroke damage to right is more likely to lead to apathy and indifference.

APHASIAS

Broca (Nonfluent)

Broca's aphasia results from lesion of frontal lobe (Brodmann area 44). Comprehension is unimpaired; speech production is telegraphic and ungrammatical.

- Often accompanied by depressive symptoms
- "I movies" instead of "I went to the movies"
- Trouble repeating statements
- Muscle weakness on the right side

Wernicke (Fluent)

Wernicke's aphasia results from lesions of superior temporal gyrus (Brodmann area 22). Comprehension is impaired; speech is fluent but incoherent.

- Trouble repeating statements
- Verbal paraphasias (substituting one word for another, or making up word)
- No muscle weakness
- Resembles formal thought disorder
- Mania-like, rapid speech hyperactivity

Conduction (Fluent)

Conduction aphasia results from a lesion in the parietal lobe or arcuate fasciculus; connection between Broca and Wernicke areas is broken. Words are comprehended correctly, but cannot be passed on for speech or writing.

- Trouble repeating statements
- Naming always impaired

Note

- Apraxia: loss of ability to learn or to carry out specific movements, e.g., unable to flip a coin when asked to do so
- Agnosia: failure to recognize sensory stimuli, e.g., visual agnosia, unable to recognize object when shown but able to recognize when touched
- Alexia: acquired disorder of reading ability; often accompanied by aphasia. Distinguish from dyslexia (developmental reading problem)
- Agraphia: acquired inability to write

Global (Nonfluent)

Global aphasia results from wide lesions in the presylvian speech area; both Broca and Wernicke areas are damaged. Includes labored telegraphic speech with poor comprehension.

- Trouble repeating statements
- Naming severely impaired

Transcortical

Transcortical aphasia results from a lesion in the prefrontal cortex; capacity to repeat statements is unimpaired. Patient cannot speak spontaneously.

BRAIN AND BEHAVIOR

Original Drawing	Patient's Drawing	Name	Localization
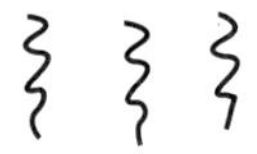	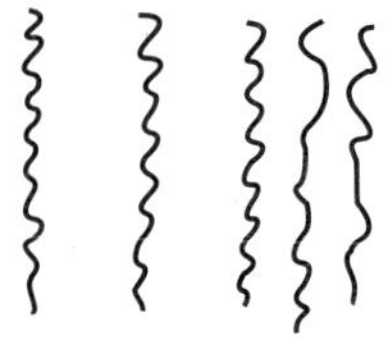	Perseveration	Frontal lobe
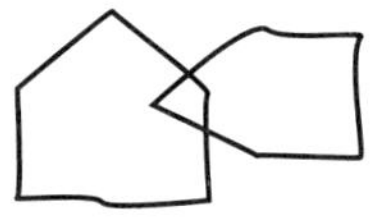	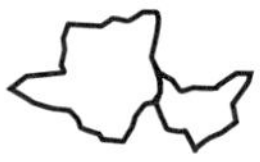	Constructional apraxia	Nondominant (right) parietal lobe
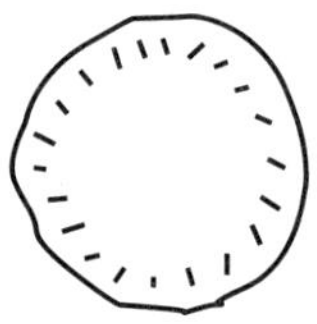	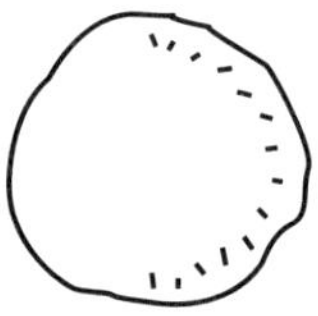	Hemineglect/ hemi-inattention	Right parietal lobe (usually non-dominant)

Figure 12-1. Dysfunctions on Common Neurologic Exams

Frontal Cortex: Global Orientation

Key functions of the frontal cortex are speech, personality, abstract thought, memory and higher-order mental functions, capacity to initiate and stop tasks, and concentration.

Lesions of dorsal prefrontal cortex:

- Apathy
- Decreased drive, initiative
- Poor grooming
- Decreased attention

- Poor ability to think abstractly
- Broca aphasia (if in dominant hemisphere)

Lesions of orbitomedial frontal cortex:

- Withdrawal
- Fearfulness
- Explosive mood
- Loss of inhibitions
- Violent outbursts

Temporal Cortex

Key functions of the temporal cortex are language, memory, and emotion. Lesions stem from stroke, tumor, and trauma; herpes virus CNS infections often affect temporal cortex.

Bilateral lesions: neurocognitive disorder

Lesions of the rostal (front) left temporal lobe: deficits in recall or learning of proper names.

Lesions of dominant lobe:

- Euphoria
- Auditory hallucinations
- Delusions
- Thought disorders
- Poor verbal comprehension (Wernicke)

Lesions of nondominant lobe:

- Dysphoria
- Irritability
- Decreased visual and musical ability

Parietal Cortex

The key function of the parietal cortex is intellectual processing of sensory information.

Left: verbal processing (dominant)

Right: visual–spatial processing (nondominant)

Lesions of dominant lobe, Gerstmann syndrome:

- Agraphia
- Acalculia
- Finger agnosia

- Right-left disorientation
- Dysfunctions in this area account for aproportion of learning disabilities

Lesions of nondominant lobe:

- Denial of illness (anosognosia)
- Construction apraxia (difficulty outlining objects)
- Neglect of the opposite side (e.g., not washing or dressing opposite side of body)

Occipital Cortex

The key functions of the occipital cortext are visual input and recall of objects, scenes, and distances; PET scans show activity in this area during recall of visual images.

- Destruction: cortical blindness
- Bilateral occlusion of posterior cerebral arteries is Anton syndrome:
  - Cortical blindness
  - Denial of blindness

Limbic System

The limbic system consists of the hippocampus, hypothalamus, anterior thalamus, cingulate gyrus, and amygdala. Associated cortical areas can suppress external displays of internal states.

Key functions are motivation, memory, emotions (mediation between cortex and lower centers), reflex arc for conditioned responses, violent behaviors, and sociosexual behaviors.

Associated dysfunctions: apathy, aggression, vegetative-endocrine disturbances, memory problems and learning new material

The **hypothalamus** is implicated in involuntary internal responses that accompany emotional strategy. Regulates some physiologic responses:

- Increased heart and respiration
- Elevation of blood pressure and diversion of blood to skeletal muscles when angry
- Regulation of endocrine balance
- Control of eating (hunger/thirst centers)
- Regulation of body temperature
- Regulation of sleep-wake cycle

Dysfunctions:

- Destruction of ventromedial hypothalamus: hyperphagia and obesity
- Destruction of lateral hypothalamus: anorexia and starvation

The **thalamus** is critical to pain perception. Dysfunctions lead to impaired memory and arousal.

The **reticular activating system (RAS)** responsible for motivation, arousal, and wakefulness.

The **hippocampus** is critical for memory and new learning.

Table 12-3. Lesions and Memory

Lesion	Short-Term Memory	Long-Term Memory	New Learning
Medial temporal lobe	Spared	Spared	Impaired
Hippocampus	Spared	Impaired	Impaired

The **amygdala** is the dorsomedial portion of temporal lobe. Connection with corpus striatum; direct link between limbic system and motor system. Plays critical role in emotional memory and rudimentary learning: the "unconscious mind"?

Klüver-Bucy syndrome: Removal of the amygdala.

- Tame
- No fear of natural enemies
- Hyperactive sexually
- High rage threshold
- "Make love, not war"

Korsakoff syndrome: Amnesia resulting from chronic thiamin deficiency; associated with alcoholism. Neuronal damage in the thalamus; once neuronal damage in the thalamus, not treatable with thiamin.

Basal Ganglia

Functions include initiation and control of movement; basal ganglia is implicated in depression and neurocognitive disorder. Dysfunctions:

- Parkinson disease
- Huntington chorea
- Wilson disease
- Fahr disease: rare hereditary disorder; calcification of the basal ganglia; onset at age 30; neurocognitive disorder at age 50; resembles negative symptom schizophrenia

Pons

The pons is the start of NE pathway; important for REM sleep. Anomalies here are linked to autism.

Cerebellum

The cerebellum is key for balance and skill-based memory and facilitates verbal recall. It is implicated in some learning disabilities.

BRIEF REVIEW OF NEUROTRANSMITTERS

Acetylcholine (ACh)

ACh is a neurotransmitter at nerve-muscle connections for all voluntary muscles of the body and also many of the involuntary (autonomic) nervous system synapses. The exact role of ACh in the brain unclear.

- Cholinergic neurons concentrated in the RAS and basal forebrain
- Significant role in Alzheimer disease
- Neurocognitive disorder in general associated with decreased ACh concentrations in amygdala, hippocampus, and temporal neocortex
- Associated with erections in males
- Muscarinic and nicotinic receptors
- In the corpus striatum, ACh circuits are in equilibrium with dopamine neurons.

Norepinephrine (NE)

NE is one of the catecholamine neurotransmitters. It is a transmitter of the sympathetic nerves of the autonomic nervous system, which mediate emergency response.

- Acceleration of the heart
- Dilatation of the bronchi
- Elevation of blood pressure

NE is implicated in altering attention, perception, and mood. The key pathway is locus ceruleus in upper pons. It is implicated in monoamine hypothesis of affective disorders:

- Depletion of NE leads to depression
- Excess of NE (and serotonin) leads to mania
- Based on 2 observations: reserpine depletes NE and causes depression; antidepressant drugs block NE re-uptake, thus increasing the amount of NE available postsynaptically

Receptors:

- Alpha-1: sympathetic (vasoconstriction)
- Alpha-2: on cell bodies of presynaptic neurons, inhibit NE release
- Beta-1: excitatory for heart, lungs, brain
- Beta-2: excitatory for vasodilatation and bronchodilatation

Dopamine

Dopamine is the other catecholamine neurotransmitter, synthesized from the amino acid tyrosine.

- D_2 receptors most important
- D_1 and D_5 stimulate G-protein and increase cAMP and excitation
- D_2, D_3, and D_4 inhibit G-protein and decrease cAMP and excitation

Three pathways of known psychiatric importance:

- Nigrostriatal pathway: Blockade leads to tremors, muscle rigidity, bradykinesia
- Meso-limbic-cortico pathway: Blockade leads to reduction of psychotic symptoms
- Tuberoinfundibular system: Blockade leads to increases in prolactin (Dop = PIF)

Serotonin (5-Hydroxytryptamine, 5-HT)

Serotonin is the transmitter of a discrete group of neurons that all have cell bodies located in the raphe nuclei of the brain stem. Changes in the activity of serotonin neurons are related to the actions of psychedelic drugs. It is involved in the therapeutic mechanism of action of antidepressant treatments (most are 5-HT re-uptake inhibitors; a few new ones are 5-HT agonists).

- Has inhibitory influence; linked to impulse control
- Low 5-HT = low impulse control
- Has role in regulation of mood, sleep, sexual activity, aggression, anxiety, motor activity, cognitive function, appetite, circadian rhythms, neuroendocrine function, and body temperature

Glutamic Acid

Glutamic acid is one of the major amino acids in general metabolism and protein synthesis; it's also a neurotransmitter. It stimulates neurons to fire and is the principal excitatory neurotransmitter in the brain and the neurotransmitter of the major neuronal pathway that connects the cerebral cortex and the corpus striatum. Glutamic acid is also the transmitter of the granule cells, which are the most numerous neurons in the cerebellum.

There is evidence that glutamic acid is the principal neurotransmitter of the visual pathway. It may have a role in producing schizophrenic symptoms; is the reason for PCP symptoms (antagonist of NMDA glutamate receptors). Glutamate agonists produce seizures in animal studies.

Enkephalins

Enkephalins are composed of 2 peptides, each containing 5 amino acids. They are normally occurring substances that act on opiate receptors, mimicking the effects of opiates. Neurons are localized to areas of the brain that regulate functions influenced by opiate drugs.

Substance P

Substance P is a peptide containing 11 amino acids and a major transmitter of sensory neurons that convey pain sensation from the periphery, especially the skin, into the spinal cord; also found in numerous brain regions. Opiates relieve pain in part by blocking the release of substance P. There is a new class of anti-depressant medications being tested to work on substance P.

Gamma Amino-butyric Acid (GABA)

GABA is one of the amino-acid transmitters in the brain. It occurs almost exclusively in the brain, reduces the firing of neurons, and is the principle inhibitory neurotransmitter in the brain. GABA is the transmitter present at 25 to 40% of all synapses in the brain; quantitatively, it is the predominant transmitter in the brain. GABA is associated with anxiety, cannabis, benzodiazepines.

Psychopharmacology 13

Learning Objectives

- ❑ Describe the pharmacokinetics, effects, side effects, and appropriate use of antipsychotics (neuroleptics), antidepressants, mood stabilizers, and anxiolytics

ANTIPSYCHOTICS (NEUROLEPTICS)

With antipsychotic medications, there are a few treatment concerns. The most common cause of relapse is **nonadherence**. The most common reason for failure of treatment is **inadequate dosage**. Keep in mind that worse behavioral symptoms are seen in those taking antipsychotics, so check for an undiagnosed organic condition.

Common uses for antipsychotic medications are:

- Psychotic symptoms: hallucinations, alterations of affect, ideas of reference, delusions, etc.
- Movement disorders: Tourette's (haloperidol, pimozide, clonidine, risperidone), Huntington, and hemiballism (flailing movements)
- Nausea and vomiting
- Intractable hiccups
- Pruritus

Mechanisms of action include:

- Dopamine blockage at postsynaptic receptors
- Alpha-adrenergic blockade; therefore, hypotensive effect
- Anticholinergic action by blocking the muscarinic receptors
- Blocks both NE re-uptake and serotonin and histamine receptors

Neurologic effects include anticholinergic effects, CNS effects, and extrapyramidal reactions.

Anticholinergic effects (very common, especially in the elderly) include dry mouth, blurry vision, constipation, urinary retention, delirium. If given with other anticholinergic agents, the effects are additive, i.e., blocks parasympathetic receptors. Also:

- **CNS effects**, from antagonism of H1 receptors, include weight gain, sedation (very common), and impaired memory.

Note

Extrapyramidal reactions:

- Choreiform: jerky movements
- Athetoid: slow, continuous movements
- Rhythmic: stereotypical movements

- **Extrapyramidal reactions**, caused by decreased dopamine, appear in 50% of all patients in the first few months. Treat with benztropine, trihexyphenidyl, diphenhydramine.
- **Tardive dyskinesia** (TD) (rarely seen earlier than 3–6 months [1 month if age >60]), caused by a supersensitivity of postsynaptic dopamine receptors
  - Signs are tongue protrusion, tremors and spasms of the neck, body, and limbs; stress and movements in other body parts will aggravate condition
  - May persist even after medication terminated (5–10% remit), incapacitating in 5% of cases
  - Predisposing factors include older age, long treatment, smoking, diabetes mellitus.
  - Symptoms do not occur during sleep
  - Suppressed by voluntary movements for short time (versus cerebellar disease tremor, which worsens with intentional movement)
  - No treatment available, so focus is on prevention: pimozide or loxapine has less chance of inducing TD, clozapine not associated with TD at all

Table 13-1. Extrapyramidal Reactions to Antipsychotic Medications

Side Effects	Peak
Dystonic reactions (jerky movements, trouble speaking)	1 week (younger are more at risk)
Akinesia	2 weeks
Rigidity	3 weeks
Tremors	6 weeks
Akathisia	10 weeks
Pisa and Rabbit syndromes	18+ weeks

Non-neurologic effects include:

- **Cardiovascular effects**: orthostatic hypotension (do not use epinephrine as it lowers blood pressure further)
- **Particular taste** (also dental cavities)
- **Vomiting**: common with long-term use, especially among smokers
- **Sexual effects**: prolactin elevated (decreased libido, inhibition of ejaculation, retrograde ejaculation [men] and breast enlargement and lactation, changes in libido [women])
- Altered bodily response to temperature

Table 13-2. Potency of Antipsychotic Medications

Potency	Extrapyramidal Symptoms	Anticholinergic Effects
High (haloperidol)	High	Low
Low (chlorpromazine)	Low	High

Table 13-3. Typical versus Atypical Antipsychotics

Typical	Atypical
Dopamine	Dopamine and serotonin
Treats mostly positive symptoms	Treats positive and negative symptoms
More side effects	Fewer side effects

Typical Anti-Psychotics

Haloperidol (Typical) and Fluphenazine (Typical)

Short- and long-acting preparations; still used frequently

Thioridazine (Typical)

Retinitis pigmentosa; retrograde ejaculation

Atypical Anti-Psychotics

Clozapine (Atypical)

Weak reaction on D2 receptors; high affinity for serotonin receptors. Affects negative and positive symptoms. Side effects are agranulocytosis (more common in Jews) (<1%) and seizures (14% of doses >600 mg). Less incidence of EP, TD, prolactin, or sexual effects.

Risperidone (Atypical)

Affects positive and negative symptoms, thought disorders. Side effects are dizziness, fatigue, dry mouth, tachycardia, hypotension. Raises prolactin levels, EP effects. Highest risk of movement disorders.

Olanzapine (Atypical)

Affects positive and negative symptoms, thought disorders. Highest incidence of diabetes. Increased weight, increased cholesterol.

Quetiapine (Atypical)

D2 and 5-HT2 antagonist; also affects H1 and alpha-1 receptors. For schizophrenia and bipolar. Side effects: somnolence, dizziness, dry mouth, weight gain. Lowest risk of movement side effects.

Aripiprazole (Atypical)

Partial agonist on D2 and 5-HT1 receptors. Antagonist at 5-HT2 receptor. Side effects: akathisia, headache, tiredness, nausea. Also used for bipolar and adjunt therapy for depression. Partial dopamine against at low doses.

Ziprasidone (Atypical)

High affinity for DA, 5-HT, alpha-adrenergic, and histamine receptors; some inhibition of 5-HT reuptake. For acute agitation of psychoses, acute mania. Intramuscular injection; prolongs QT interval.

ANTIDEPRESSANTS

Antidepressants are used for depression, anxiety, chronic pain (with and without depression).

Cyclic Antidepressants

Action: blocking of re-uptake of serotonin and norepinephrine, blocking of alpha-1 adrenergic receptors, and muscarinic receptors.

Pharmacokinetics: fat soluble; metabolized by the liver and excreted by the kidneys; requires reaching plasma levels for imipramine, nortriptyline, desipramine, and amitriptyline for efficacy.

Anticholinergic effects: (see Antipsychotics section)

CNS effects: drowsiness, insomnia and agitation, disorientation and confusion, headache, fine tremor

Cardiovascular effects: from antagonism of alpha-1 adrenoreceptors and inhibition of 5-HT reuptake

- Most common in elderly
- Tachycardia
- Orthostatic hypotension: managed by sodium chloride tablets, caffeine, support hose, or biofeedback
- Lethal in overdose due to cardiac complications

Sexual effects: men: impotence, testicular swelling; women: anorgasmia and breast enlargement (treat with cyproheptadine)

Metabolic effects: changes in blood sugar levels

Cautions:

- Effective in only 70% of depressed patients
- Not for patients with respiratory difficulties; dries up bronchial secretions
- May lower seizure threshold
- May impair driving
- Potentiates effects of alcohol
- Manic episode induced in 50% of bipolars
- Avoid during first trimester; baby gets 1% of mother's dose in breast milk

Withdrawal: After prolonged use, withdrawal should be gradual; akathisia, dyskinesia, anxiety, sweating, dizziness, vomiting, cholinergic rebound, depression rebound

Selective Serotonin Reuptake Inhibitors (SSRIs)

SSRIs are the most widely used antidepressants. They have no effect on NE or dopamine, and very selective blockage of reuptake of serotonin. They have the fewest adverse effects of any antidepressants currently available.

Adverse effects:

- **Anorgasmia and delayed orgasm** (15–20% of patients)
- **Serotonin syndrome** (associated with high doses, MAOI/SSRI combo, MAOI/synthetic narcotic combo
  - Symptoms: general restlessness, sweating, insomnia, nausea, diarrhea, cramps, delirium
  - Treatment: remove causative agent, stop SSRIs, give cyproheptadine

Drugs from this class:

- Fluoxetine: longest half-life
- Sertraline
- Paroxetine
- Fluvoxamine: approved for OCD
- Citalopram
- Escitalopram

Monoamine Oxidase Inhibitors (MAOIs)

MAOIs inhibits MAO, an enzyme that metabolizes serotonin, epinephrine, and NE. For the best effect, reduce MAO activity by 80%.

MAOI + tyramine = Hypertensive Crisis

- Problem foods: cheese, dried fish, sauerkraut, sausage, chocolate, avocados
- Safe foods: cottage cheese, some wines
- Signs: occipital headache, stiff neck, nausea and vomiting, chest pain, dilated pupils, nosebleed, elevated blood pressure
- Treatment: stop medication, give phentolamine (alpha-blockage) or chlorpromazine (antipsychotic with hypotensive effects)

Electroconvulsive Therapy

Electroconvulsive therapy (ECT) is used for depression (80%), schizoaffective disorder (10%), and bipolar disorder. Electricity is passed from the frontal cortex to the striatum, with 5–10 treatments usually required. Around 90% show some immediate improvement. The only relative contraindication is increased cranial pressure (e.g., tumor).

Side effects of ECT include memory loss and headache (common); patient returns to normal in several weeks. Serious complications <1:1,000.

Although not usually first-line treatment, ECT should be considered for highly suicidal patients and depressed pregnant patients. Improvement is associated with a large increase in slow wave (delta) activity in the prefrontal area, i.e., greater increase = greater recovery.

Drugs to Highlight

Trazodone

5-HT receptor antagonist, alpha-1 blocker. Almost no anticholinergic adverse effects. Sedating, but effective at improving sleep quality, does not decrease Stage 4 sleep. May lead to priapism; therefore, sometimes used to treat erectile dysfunction.

Mirtazapine

Stimulates NE and 5-HT release; blocks 5-HT2 and 5-HT3 receptors. Side effects: somnolence (60%), increased appetite, weight gain.

Bupropion

Weak inhibitor of dopamine, modest effect on NE, no effect on 5-HT reuptake. No anticholinergic effect; little cardiac depressant effect. Increased risk of seizures. Less sexual effects or weight gain. Side effects: appetite suppressant, agitation, insomnia. Approved for smoking cessation.

Venlafaxine

Inhibits reuptake of NE and 5-HT, mild dopamine effect (SNRI). Side effects: sweating, nausea, constipation, anorexia, vomiting, somnolence, tremor, impotence.

Duloxetine

Targets 5-HT and NE receptors (SNRI). Side effects: nausea, dry mouth, dizziness, constipation, decreased appetite, increased blood pressure. Approved for depression and neuropathic pain

MOOD STABILIZERS

Lithium

Lithium is used for long-term control and prophylaxis of bipolar disorder, migraine cluster headaches, and chronic aggression. It is combined with tricyclics for resistant depression (effective for 70% of cases). The hypothesized mechanism of action of lithium is that it blocks inositol-1-phosphate (second messenger).

Lithium is quickly absorbed from the GI tract, not protein bound or metabolized; it requires reaching plasma levels very close to toxic levels for full effect, which is reached in 10–14 days. Blood levels must be monitored.

- Therapeutic levels: 0.8–1.5 mEq/L
- 1.4 mEq/L may be toxic
- Frank toxicity at 2.0; if >2.5, hemodialysis

Good kidney function and adequate salt and fluid intake are essential with lithium; 95% is excreted in urine with peak serum level at 1–3 hours. Potassium-sparing diuretics have no effect; loop diuretics will produce increased serum levels.

Side effects:

- Narrow margin of safety, must monitor blood levels
- Tremor, thirst, anorexia, gastrointestinal distress commonly occur at therapeutic levels
- Seizures and coma
- Polyuria and polydipsia
- Edema
- Acne
- Benign leukocytosis
- Hypothyroidism
- Nephrotoxic
- Diabetes insipidus
- Long-term lithium use has adverse effects on renal function.
- Compliance often difficult, patient may value manic experiences
- Teratogenic, produces cardiac malformations (Ebstein anomaly tricuspid valve)

Valproic Acid

For acute mania, rapid cycling bipolar disorder, impulse control. Mechanism of action is augmentation of GABA in CNS. Monitor blood levels, as it can be hepatotoxic (liver function impaired).

Side effects:

- Sedation
- Mild tremor
- Gastrointestinal distress
- Occasional agranulocytosis
- At toxic levels: confusion, coma, cardiac arrest
- Teratogenic (neural tube defect)

Carbamazepine: Second-line Treatment

For acute mania, rapid cycling bipolar disorder, impulse control. Mechanism of action: blocks sodium channels in neurons with action potential; alters central GABA receptors; monitors blood levels and signs of rash.

Side effects:

- Similar to valproic acid, plus nausea, rash, mild leukopenia
- Occasional agranulocytosis
- Aplastic anemia
- Toxic levels: atrioventricular block, respiratory depression, coma

ANXIOLYTICS (ANTIANXIETY)

Benzodiazepines

Benzodiazepines are used for anxiety, acute and chronic alcohol withdrawal, convulsions, insomnia, "restless legs," akathisia, and panic disorder. They work by depressing the CNS at the limbic system, RAS, and cortex. They bind to GABA-chloride receptors, facilitating the action of GABA.

All benzodiazepines undergo hepatic microsomal oxidation, except for lorazepam, oxazepam, and temazepam, which undergo glucuronide conjugation. They are well-absorbed orally.

Adverse effects:

- CNS depression (sedative effect)
- Paradoxical agitation
- Confusion and disorientation, especially in elderly
- Overdose: apnea and respiratory depression (not for use with patients with sleep apnea)
- Withdrawal: insomnia, agitation, anxiety rebound, gastrointestinal distress; abrupt withdrawal can bring on seizures

Diminishes effectiveness of ECT. Lowers tolerance to alcohol. Crosses placenta and accumulates in fetus, withdrawal symptoms in newborn; passed on in breast milk with observable effects. Oral contraceptives decrease metabolism of benzodiazepines.

Buspirone

Buspirone is used for anxiety. It has no anticonvulsant or muscle-relaxing properties. It works by affecting serotonin, not GABA. Full effect is seen >7 days. Some sedation is seen. It has no withdrawal effect and is not potentiated by alcohol. It has low-abuse potential.

Review Questions

1. Following his arrest for disturbing the peace, a 35-year-old man is referred for psychiatric evaluation. During the initial interview, he talks rapidly and paces around the room. He reports that he has slept little in the past few days, but that he feels "great." "It's not always like this," he confides. "Sometimes I just feel so bad I can hardly move." During the most common subsequent treatment for this disorder, the patient will most likely experience which of the following side effects?

   A. Insomnia

   B. Memory loss

   C. Tardive dyskinesia

   D. Acne

   E. Retarded ejaculation

2. A 36-year-old woman is brought to her physician by a family member, who reports that over the past year she has had trouble controlling her movements. Symptoms include frequent and discrete brisk movements that cause jerks of the pelvis and limbs as well as facial frowns, grimaces, and smirks. The most likely diagnosis for this patient would be

   A. Pick disease

   B. Wilson disease

   C. Parkinson disease

   D. Huntington disease

   E. Creutzfeldt-Jakob disease

3. Over a 5-week period, a previously healthy 55-year-old woman develops headaches, progressively severe word-finding difficulty, and confusion. She speaks incoherently and is unable to follow commands, repeat phrases, or name objects. What is the most likely site of the lesion?

   A. Frontal lobe

   B. Temporal lobe

   C. Occipital lobe

   D. Parietal lobe

   E. Cerebellum

4. Following a car accident, a 46-year-old man is brought to the hospital with head trauma. Over the next week, his medical record notes the appearance of auditory hallucinations, delusions, thought disorders, and poor verbal comprehension. These symptoms are most consistent with a lesion in the

   A. frontal lobe

   B. dominant parietal lobe

   C. nondominant parietal lobe

   D. dominant temporal lobe

   E. nondominant temporal lobe

5. A 32-year-old man presents at the local clinic complaining of abdominal cramps, sweating, runny nose, vomiting, and muscle aches. Examination shows that his pulse is rapid and pupils are dilated. He states that he feels "just awful" and that he has had these symptoms for about 24 hours. The most likely pharmacologic treatment would be

   A. none
   B. diazepam
   C. carbamazepine
   D. clonidine
   E. trazodone

6. A 58-year-old chronic alcoholic is evaluated and found to have difficulty with recall of recent events although long-term memories seem intact. He appears confused and insists he has met the physician before, though that is not accurate. These symptoms are the result of a syndrome that can result from neuronal damage to the

   A. cerebellum
   B. hippocampus
   C. hypothalamus
   D. reticular activating system
   E. thalamus

7. A 32-year-old schizophrenic man has been taking a standard course of neuroleptic medication for the past year. The medication has been very effective at controlling his delusions and hallucinations. However, during a regular checkup he is found to be suffering from dry mouth and constipation. The patient reports that it is hard to read because his vision is blurry, and then lapses into delirium. These symptoms are most likely produced by blockage of what receptors?

   A. Dopamine
   B. Histamine
   C. Muscarinic
   D. Norepinephrine
   E. Serotonin

8. A 24-year-old woman is diagnosed with undifferentiated schizophrenia and placed on a standard drug regimen. About 2 weeks into her treatment, she experiences disturbing extrapyramidal side effects. The most likely side effect to appear at this time would be

   A. akathisia
   B. akinesia
   C. physical tremors
   D. Pisa syndrome
   E. tardive dyskinesia

9. Patients placed on which of the following medications most likely should have blood drawn and checked on a weekly basis?

    A. Clozapine
    B. Haloperidol
    C. Olanzapine
    D. Risperidone
    E. Thioridazine

10. A 46-year-old man who was being treated for depression is brought to the emergency department complaining of headache at the base of the skull, chest pains, and stiff neck. Physical exam shows that his nose is bleeding, his pupils are dilated, and his blood pressure is extremely high. He reports vomiting repeatedly in the past few hours. Based on this initial presentation, the physician suspects that the patient has recently eaten which of the following foods?

    A. Avocados
    B. Cottage cheese
    C. Hamburger
    D. Raw eggs
    E. French fries
    F. Fried chicken
    G. Dried figs

Answers and Explanations

1. **Answer: D.** Lithium has been associated with side effects leading to lethargy (hypothyroidism), edema (lithium is a salt), acne, and seizures.

2. **Answer: D.** Age of onset and description indicate the onset of Huntington chorea.

3. **Answer: B.** The temporal lobe is associated with language, memory, and emotional expression.

4. **Answer: D.** Lesions of the dominant temporal lobe result in euphoria, auditory hallucinations, thought disorder, and poor verbal comprehension.

5. **Answer: D.** The man is suffering from opiate withdrawal. The drug on the list to treat the withdrawal is clonidine.

6. **Answer: E.** The man most likely is suffering from Korsakoff syndrome, in which chronic thiamin deficiency leads to neuronal damage in the thalamus as well as the frontal lobes.

7. **Answer: C.** The patient displays the symptoms of anticholinergic intoxication. This is the result of blockage of the muscarinic receptors.

8. **Answer: B.** Difficulty completing simple movements or common skills occurs relatively early in the course of treatment. Tremors and akathisia appear after 1 to 2 months. Tardive dyskinesia rarely occurs before the patient is on the medication for at least 3 months.

9. **Answer: A.** Because of the risk of agranulocytosis with clozapine, blood must be monitored weekly.

10. **Answer: A.** The patient is suffering from a hypertensive crisis, likely the result of consuming tyramine-containing food while on MAOIs for his depression. Tyramine can be acquired from cheese, dried fish, sauerkraut, sausage, chocolate, or avocados.

Ethical and Legal Issues 14

Learning Objectives

- ❑ Demonstrate understanding of selected important court cases
- ❑ Differentiate between legal issues and ethical issues as they are related to medical practice

SELECTED IMPORTANT COURT CASES

Karen Ann Quinlan: Substituted Judgment Standard

In the Quinlan case, Karen Ann was in a persistent vegetative state, being kept alive only by life support. Karen's father asked to have her life support terminated according to his understanding of what Karen Ann would want. The court found that "if Karen herself were miraculously lucid for an interval . . . and perceptive of her irreversible condition, she could effectively decide upon discontinuance of the life support apparatus, even if it meant the prospect of natural death."

The court therefore allowed termination of life support, not because the father asked, but because it held that the father's request was most likely the expression of Karen Ann's own wishes.

Substituted judgment begins with the premise that decisions belong to the competent patient by virtue of the rights of autonomy and privacy. In this case, however, the patient is unable to decide, and a decision-maker who is the best representative of the patient's wishes must be substituted. In legal terms, the patient has the right to decide but is incompetent to do so. Therefore, the decision is made for the patient on the basis of the best estimate of his or her subjective wishes.

Note the key here is *not* who is the closest next of kin, but who is most likely to represent the patient's own wishes.

Brother Fox *(Eichner vs Dillon)*: Best Interest Standard

The New York Court of Appeals, in its decision of *Eichner vs Dillon,* held that trying to determine what a never-competent patient would have decided is practically impossible. Obviously, it is difficult to ascertain the actual (subjective) wishes of incompetents. Therefore, if the patient has always been incompetent, or no one knows the patient well enough to render substituted judgment, the use of substituted judgment standard is questionable, at best.

Under these circumstances, decisions are made for the patient using the **best interest standard**, the object of which is to decide what a hypothetical "reasonable person" would decide after weighing the benefits and burdens of each course of action.

Note here the issue of who makes the decision is less important. All persons applying the best-interest standard should come to the same conclusions.

Infant Doe: Foregoing Lifesaving Surgery, Parents Withholding Treatment

As a general rule, parents cannot withhold life- or limb-saving treatment from their children. Yet, in this exceptional case they did.

Baby Boy Doe was born with Down syndrome (trisomy 21) and with a tracheoesophageal fistula. The infant's parents were informed that surgery to correct his fistula would have "an even chance of success." Left untreated, the fistula would soon lead to the infant's death from starvation or pneumonia. The parents, who also had two healthy children, chose to withhold food and treatment and "let nature take its course."

Court action to remove the infant from his parents' custody (and permit the surgery) was sought by the county prosecutor. The court denied such action, and the Indiana Supreme Court declined to review the lower court's ruling. Infant Doe died at 6 days of age, as Indiana authorities were seeking intervention from the U.S. Supreme Court.

Note that this case is simply an application of the best-interest standard. The court agreed with the parents that the burdens of treatment far outweighed any expected benefits.

Roe vs Wade (1973): The Patient Decides

Known to most people as the "abortion legalizing decision," the importance of this case is not limited to its impact on abortion. Faced with a conflict between the rights of the mother and the rights of the putative unborn child, the court held that in the first trimester, the mother's rights are paramount, and that states may, if they wish, have the mother's rights remain paramount for the full term of the pregnancy. Because the mother gets to decide, even in the face of threats to the fetus, by extension, all patients get to decide about their own bodies and the health care they receive. In the United States, the locus for decision-making about health care resides with the patient, not the physician.

Note that courts have held that a pregnant woman has the right to refuse care (e.g., blood transfusions) even if it places her unborn child at risk.

Tarasoff Decision: Duty to Warn and Duty to Protect

A student visiting a counselor at a counseling center in California states that he is going to kill someone. When he leaves, the counselor is concerned enough to call the police but takes no further action. The student subsequently kills the person he threatened. The court found the counselor and the center liable because they did not go far enough to warn and protect the potential victim.

The counselor should have called the police and then should also have tried in every way possible to notify the potential victim of the potential danger.

In similar situations, first try to detain the person making the threat, next call the police, and finally notify and warn the potential victim. All 3 actions should be taken, or at least attempted.

LEGAL ISSUES RELATED TO MEDICAL PRACTICE

This section lays out a set of rules that constitute the general consensus of legal opinion. Apply these rules to individual situations as they arise.

Rule #1: Competent patients have the right to refuse medical treatment. Incompetent patients have the same rights, but must be exercised differently (via a surrogate). Patients have an almost absolute right to refuse. Patients have almost absolute control over their own bodies. The sicker the patient, the lesser the chance of recovery, the greater the right to refuse treatment.

Note

Family matters only to the degree that reflects the patient's wishes. Family's own wishes are not relevant.

Rule #2: If patient is incompetent to make decisions, physician may rely on advance directives. Advance directives can be oral. Living will is a written document expressing wishes. Care facilities must provide information at time of admission; responsibility of the institution, not the physician. Only applies to end-of-life care.

Health power of attorney: designating the surrogate decision-maker

- "Speaks with the patient's voice"
- Beats all other decision rules
- In end-of-life circumstances, if power of attorney person *directly* contradicts the living will, follow the living will.

Rule #3: Assume that the patient is competent unless clear behavioral evidence indicates otherwise. Competence is a legal, not a medical issue; a diagnosis, by itself, tells you little about a patient's competence. Clear behavioral evidence:

- Patient is grossly psychotic and dysfunctional
- Patient's physical or mental state prevents simple communication

If you are unsure, assume the patient is competent. The patient does not have to prove to you that he is competent. You have to have clear evidence to assume that he is not.

Rule #4: When surrogates make decisions for a patient, they should use the following criteria and in this order:

1. Subjective standard: actual intent, advance directive; What did the patient say in the past?
2. Substituted judgment: Who best represents the patient? What would patient say if he or she could?
3. Best-interest standard: burdens vs. benefits; interests of patient, not preferences of the decision-maker

Rule #5: Feeding tube is a medical treatment and can be withdrawn at the patient's request. Not considered killing the patient, but stopping treatment at patient's request. A competent person can refuse even lifesaving hydration and nutrition.

Rule #6: Do nothing to actively assist the patient to die sooner. Active euthanasia and assisted suicide are on difficult ground.

- Passive, i.e., allowing to die = OK
- Active, i.e., killing = NOT OK

On the other hand, do all you can to reduce the patient's suffering (e.g., giving pain medication).

Rule #7: The physician decides when the patient is dead. If the physician thinks continued treatment is futile (the patient has shown no improvement), but the surrogate insists on continued treatment, the treatment should continue. If there are no more treatment options (the patient is cortically dead), and the family insists on treatment, there is nothing the physician can do; treatment must stop.

Rule #8: Never abandon a patient. Lack of financial resources or lack of results are never reasons to stop treatment of a patient. An annoying or difficult patient is still your patient. You cannot ever threaten abandonment.

Rule #9: Keep the physician–patient relationship within bounds. Intimate social contact with anyone who is or has been a patient is prohibited. AMA guidelines say, "for at least 2 years." Do not date parents of pediatric patients or children of geriatric patients. Do not treat friends or family. Do not prescribe for colleagues unless a physician/patient relationship exists. If patients are inappropriate, gently but clearly let them know what acceptable behavior would be. Any gift from a patient beyond a small token should be declined.

Rule #10 Stop harm from happening. Beyond "do no harm," you must stop anyone from hurting himself or others. Take whatever action is required to prevent harm. Harm can be spreading disease, physical assault, psychological abuse, neglect, infliction of pain or anything which produces notable distress. You must also protect your patient, or anyone not your patient, from being hurt by another.

Rule #11: Always obtain informed consent. Full, informed consent requires that the patient has received and understood 5 pieces of information:

- Nature of procedure
- Purpose or rationale
- Benefits
- Risks
- Availability of alternatives

There are 4 exceptions to informed consent:

- Emergency
- Waiver by patient
- Patient is incompetent
- Therapeutic privilege (unconscious, confused, physician deprives patient of autonomy in interest of health)

Gag clauses that prohibit a physician from discussing treatment options that are not approved violate informed consent and are illegal. Consent can be oral. A signed paper the patient has not read or does not understand does NOT constitute informed consent. Written consent can be revoked orally at any time.

Rule #12: Special rules apply with children. Children younger than 18 years are minors and are legally incompetent. Exceptions are emancipated minors:

- If older than 13 years and taking care of self, i.e., living alone, treat as an adult.
- Marriage makes a child emancipated, as does serving in the military.
- Pregnancy or giving birth, in most cases, does not.

For partial emancipation, many states have special ages of consent: generally age 14 and older for certain issues only:

- Substance drug treatment
- Prenatal care
- Sexually transmitted disease treatment
- Birth control

Rule #13: Parents cannot withhold life- or limb-saving treatment from their children. If parents refuse permission to treat child, if immediate emergency, go ahead and treat; if not immediate, but still critical (e.g., juvenile diabetes), generally the child is declared a ward of the court and the court grants permission. If not life- or limb-threatening (e.g., child needs minor stitches), listen to the parents.

Note that the child cannot give permission. A child's refusal of treatment is irrelevant.

Rule #14: For the purposes of the exam, issues governed by laws that vary widely across states cannot be tested. This includes elective abortions (minor and spousal rights differ by locality) and legal age for drinking alcohol (varies by state).

Rule #15: Good Samaritan Laws limit liability in nonmedical settings.

- Not required to stop to help
- If help offered, shielded from liability provided:
  - Actions are within physician's competence
  - Only accepted procedures are performed.
  - Physician remains at scene after starting therapy until relieved by competent personnel
  - No compensation changes hands

Rule #16: Confidentiality is absolute. Physicians cannot tell anyone anything about their patient without the patient's permission. Physician must strive to ensure that others *cannot* access patient information. Getting a consultation is permitted, as the consultant is bound by confidentiality, too. However, watch the location of the consultation. Be careful not to be overheard (e.g., in an elevator or cafeteria). If you receive a court subpoena, show up in court but do not divulge information about your patient. If patient is a threat to self or other, the physician MUST break confidentiality:

- Duty to warn and duty to protect (Tarasoff case)
- A specific threat to a specific person
- Suicide, homicide, and abuse are obvious threats.
- Infectious disease should generally be treated as a threat, but be careful. Here issue is usually getting the patient to work with you to tell the person who is at risk
- In the case of an STD, the issue is not really whether to inform a sexual partner, but how they should be told. Best advice: Have patient and partner come to your office.

Rule #17: Patients should be given the chance to state DNR (Do Not Resuscitate) orders, and physicians should follow them. DNR refers only to cardiopulmonary resuscitation, so continue with ongoing treatments. Most physicians are unaware of DNR orders; DNR decisions are made by the patient or surrogate. Have DNR discussions as part of your first encounter with the patient. Explain details of what is entailed. Repeated discussion are not necessary.

Rule #18: Committed mentally ill patients retain their rights. Committed mentally ill adults legally are entitled to the following:

- They must have treatment available.
- They can refuse treatment.
- They can command a jury trial to determine "sanity".
- They lose only the civil liberty to come and go.
- They retain their competence for conducting business transactions, marriage, divorce, voting, driving

The words "sanity" and "competence" are legal, not psychiatric, terms. They refer to prediction of dangerousness, and medicopsychological studies show that health care professionals cannot reliably and validly predict such dangerousness.

Rule #19: Detain patients to protect them or others. Emergency detention can be effected by a physician and/or a law enforcement person for 48 hours, pending a hearing. A physician can detain; only a judge can commit. With children, special rules exist. Children can be committed only if:

- They are in imminent danger to self and/or others.
- They are unable to care for their own daily needs.
- The parents have absolutely no control over the child, and the child is in danger (e.g., fire-setter), but not because the parents are unwilling to discipline a child.

Rule #20: Remove from patient contact health care professionals who pose risk to patients. Types of risks include infectious disease (TB), substance-related disorders, depression (or other psychological issues), incompetence. Insist that they take time off; contact their supervisors if necessary. The patient, not professional solidarity, comes first.

Rule #21: Focus on what is the best ethical conduct, not simply the letter of the law. The best answers are those that are both legal and ethical.

Consider the following questions.

- Should physicians answer questions from insurance companies or employers? (Not without a release from the patient)
- Should physicians answer questions from the patient's family without the patient's explicit permission? (No)
- What information can the physician withhold from the patient? (Nothing. If patient may react negatively, figure out how to tell patient to mitigate negative outcome)
- What if the family requests that certain information be kept from the patient? (Tell the patient, but first find out why they don't want the patient told)
- Who owns the medical record? (Health care provider, but patient must be given access or copy upon request)

What should the physician do in each of these situations?

- Patient refuses lifesaving treatment on religious grounds? (Don't treat)
- Wife refuses to consent to emergency lifesaving treatment for unconscious husband citing religious grounds? (Treat, no time to assess substituted judgment)
- Wife produces card stating unconscious husband's wish to not be treated on religious grounds? (Don't treat)
- Mother refuses to consent to emergency lifesaving treatment for her daughter on religious grounds? (Treat)
- What if the child's life is at risk, but the risk is not immediate? (Court takes guardianship)
- From whom do you get permission to treat a girl who is 17 years old? (Her guardian)

From whom does the physician obtain consent in each case?

- A 17-year-old girl's parents are out of the country and the girl is staying with a babysitter? (If a threat to health, the physician can treat under doctrine of *in locum parentis*)
- A 17-year-old girl who has been living on her own and taking care of herself? (The girl herself)
- A 17-year-old girl who is married? (The girl herself)
- A 17-year-old girl who is pregnant? (Her guardian)
- A 16-year-old daughter refuses medication but her mother consents, do you write the prescription? (Yes)
- The 16-year-old daughter consents, but the mother refuses? (No)
- The mother of a minor consents, but the father refuses? (Only one permission needed)
- When should the physician provide informed consent? (Always)

- Must informed consent be written? (No)
- Can written consent be revoked orally? (Yes)
- Can you get informed consent from a schizophrenic man? (Yes, unless there is clear behavioral evidence that he is incompetent)
- Must you get informed consent from a prisoner if the police bring in the prisoner for examination? (Yes)

Review Questions

1. A 7-year-old girl is brought to the hospital by a woman who has been entrusted with her care while the girl's parents are in Mexico for vacation. The girl has sustained a non-life-threatening but serious injury during play that has almost completely severed one of her fingers from her left hand. The consensus of the physicians is that with prompt action the finger can be reattached with minimal permanent loss of movement for the child. Without prompt action, the use of the finger is likely to be lost. However, the attending physician is concerned about proceeding without the permission of the parents. The best course of action would be to

    A. try to contact the parents to get their permission to perform the procedure

    B. seek a legal injunction allowing the operation

    C. operate at once, citing the doctrine of therapeutic privilege

    D. seek the consent for the operation from the woman in whose care the girl was left

    E. seek further confirmation from additional specialists in this type of surgery

2. During the second year of residency training, you discover that the chief resident on your rotation is using amphetamines on a regular basis in order to stay alert when on call. When you mention your concern to the resident, he tells you, "Mind your own business. I'm not one of your patients." At this point, your best action would be to

    A. monitor the chief resident over the next few weeks to be sure that there is no danger to patient care

    B. talk with other residents and see if they share your concern

    C. contact the hospital ethics committee for advice and guidance

    D. contact the American Medical Association

    E. seek legal counsel

    F. schedule a meeting to speak with the residency program director

    G. lodge a complaint with the state licensing board

    H. ask the nursing staff if they have noticed anything unusual about the chief resident

3. While riding the hospital elevator to visit one of his patients, an internal medicine physician overhears two residents discussing a surgical case. The case involves a 45-year-old male who received a lymph node biopsy. The biopsy was negative. However, during the procedure, the resident performing the surgery nicked the large intestine. The mistake was noticed and quickly corrected. The resident was overheard to say, "It's all taken care of. We didn't think we needed to worry the patient by mentioning this little glitch." After overhearing this conversation, what action should the physician take?

   A. Ask the nurse for the patient's chart to confirm that the mistake was benign
   B. File a formal complaint with the hospital ethics committee
   C. File a formal complaint with the state licensing board
   D. Look up the patient and check on how he is doing
   E. Reprimand the residents on the spot and demand to speak with their supervisor
   F. No harm was done, the physician need do nothing
   G. Speak with the chairman of internal medicine
   H. Speak with the chairman of surgery
   I. Tell the residents that they need to inform the patient and suggest the best method to have the discussion

4. A 42-year-old woman has an annual physical exam, including a mammogram. She announces with great excitement that she will be getting married in 3 months and invites her physician to attend the wedding. A week later, the results of the mammogram reveal a previously undetected mass. At this point, what action should the physician take?

   A. Call the patient immediately and inform her of the findings of the mammogram
   B. Have a nurse with experience in this area call the patient and discuss the findings
   C. Make an appointment to discuss the mammogram finding with the patient within a week of receiving the results
   D. Postpone informing the patient of the findings until after the wedding so as not to upset her
   E. Schedule the patient for a confirmatory mammogram after the wedding
   F. Schedule an appointment to discuss the findings with the patient and her fiancé before the wedding

5. A 68-year-old man is seen by his physician for a monthly appointment to monitor his diabetes. The physician provides encouragement with his diet and adjusts his medication dosage. Several days later, the patient's wife telephones the physician and asks about her husband's condition and what she should do to keep him on his diet. What action should the physician take?

    A. Have the nursing staff call her back and explain the dietary regime
    B. Give her an internet address where information about diabetes can be found
    C. Obtain permission from her husband before discussing his diabetes with her
    D. Schedule an appointment to discuss the issues she raises face-to-face
    E. Ask her if her husband requested that she call
    F. Offer her a referral to another physician so she can be checked for diabetes

6. A 75-year-old man is diagnosed with severe blockage in several cardiac arteries. The standard procedure for such cases is bypass surgery that has a high rate of success. Pharmacologic options are also available, but at best will merely maintain the patient and will not remove the life-threatening blockage. Life expectancy for the pharmacologic intervention is substantially shorter than the surgical one. When presented with these available treatment options and the associated life expectancies, the patient declines the surgery and wants to be treated by pharmacologic means. The physician strongly disagrees with the patient's decision. Faced with this decision, the physician's next course of action should be to

    A. meet with the patient's family and try to convince them to change the patient's mind
    B. review the treatment options again with the patient and tell him to take a week to think it over
    C. schedule the patient for a consultation with a colleague and ask the colleague to advise the patient to choose the surgery
    D. schedule the patient for psychological evaluation
    E. start the pharmacological treatment
    F. tell the patient that you cannot agree with his choice, and cannot continue to be his physician if he insists on it
    G. tell the patient that you are required to select the treatment option with the best outcome and schedule him for surgery

7. A 54-year-old man, who makes his living as a bus driver, was sent by his company for a physical exam. The physical exam turns up nothing abnormal, although the man reports ongoing fatigue. When questioned in detail, the man professes no difficulty going to sleep. In fact, he often finds himself nodding off during the day. He also reports hallucinations as he is falling asleep and sometimes is unable to move when he wakes up in the morning. The physician suspects that the man suffers from a sleep disorder. When informed of this diagnosis, the patient requests that this information be kept confidential from his employer. At this point, the physician's best course of action is to

   A. arrange for pharmacologic treatment for the patient and maintain his confidentiality
   B. do not inform the employer, but negotiate with the patient to take time off from work on medical leave pending outcome of treatment
   C. inform his employer of his diagnosis and begin treatment
   D. refer him to a local sleep center for full evaluation and inform the employer based on the results of this workup
   E. try to obtain the patient's permission to inform the employer and schedule him for treatment
   F. schedule him for a psychiatric consult to rule out malingering

8. A 66-year-old man recently diagnosed as having prostate cancer is scheduled for an appointment to discuss his treatment options. The attending physician designates a second-year resident to meet with the patient and to obtain informed consent before proceeding with treatment. The resident meets with the patient and returns with signed informed consent forms, indicating that the patient has elected the radiation option to treat his cancer. Reviewing the conversation with the resident, the attending physician discovers that the resident did not mention a relatively new surgical procedure as a possible treatment option. At this point, what action should the attending physician take?

   A. Convene a seminar of all residents in this rotation and review the informed consent rules
   B. Exclude the resident from obtaining informed consent from patients until he has reviewed the informed consent rules
   C. Have all of the residents on the rotation accompany you while you visit the patient and demonstrate the right way to obtain informed consent
   D. Informed consent has been obtained, but instruct the resident that in the future he should mention the surgical procedure as an option to the patient
   E. Informed consent has been obtained; schedule the patient for the radiation treatment to which he has consented
   F. Instruct the resident to go back and talk to the patient again, this time mentioning the new surgical procedure
   G. Visit the patient personally and obtain informed consent again, this time mentioning the new surgical procedure

Answers and Explanations

1. **Answer: C.** The physician may exercise therapeutic privilege and assume *in locum parentis* responsibility.

2. **Answer: F.** The program director has the authority and responsibility to address the substance use issues.

3. **Answer: I.** The dual goals of training the residents and making sure the patient gets the information need to be met here. The issue is not to reprimand, but to better teach the residents.

4. **Answer: C.** *You* need to deliver the bad news, in a timely manner, and in person.

5. **Answer: C.** Confidentiality is absolute. You are not to discuss the case with her without the husband's explicit permission.

6. **Answer: E.** The patient makes medical decisions, not the physician. The options and consequences have been explained and the patient has made his choice. Begin treatment. Note that the surgical option is still available should the patient change his mind.

7. **Answer: C.** The patient likely suffers from narcolepsy, which can be debilitating and certainly makes him dangerous behind the wheel of a bus. There is a clear risk, so confidentiality must be breached to prevent harm. This is not a negotiation with the patient. The physician is obligated to act.

8. **Answer: F.** Patients must be told about all available options for informed consent to be valid. The resident should complete the job he started and go back to talk to the patient again. Getting the attending physician involved complicates the relationship with the patient and undermines the resident's confidence for handling this and similar situations.

Health Care Delivery Systems 15

Learning Objectives

- ❑ Answer questions about nongovernment and government methods of payment for services

NONGOVERNMENT METHODS OF PAYMENT FOR SERVICES

In **fee-for-service**, payment is rendered after service is delivered. The economic incentive is to do more so more can be billed; physicians make money when more treatment is provided. The danger is overtreatment.

In **standard insurance (indemnity insurance)**, the insurance company helps patient pay for health care in exchange for a periodic payment by patient (*premium*) and patient shares in payment by means of:

- **Deductible:** patient pays a certain amount before insurance assistance begins. In an annual deductible, patient pays certain amount each year; in a per-occurrence deductible, patient pays certain amount each time services are rendered.
- **Copayment:** remainder of bill is divided between patient and insurance company. Copayment calculation takes place only after deductible is satisfied. Common copayments may be patient 20%/insurance 80% or patient 30%/insurance 70%.
- **Blue Cross Blue Shield** is a nonprofit insurance company. Blue Cross covers hospital charges and physician services; coverage comes with deductibles and copayments. Premiums are intended to cover only benefits, administrative costs, and catastrophic losses.

A **health maintenance organization (HMO)** is a prepaid group practice that either hires physicians or contracts with physicians to provide services. Payment is made by **capitation**: a fixed payment is made each month. Physicians are paid for the number of patients they are responsible for, not for how much they do for each patient. The same payment is made whether services are used or not; no additional (or only minimal) payment is made when services *are* used. Physicians make money when patients stay well and do not need to use services.

Incentives:

- Under treatment
- More likely to foster preventive medicine

Table 15-1. Types of HMOs

Type	Payment to Physicians	Who owns Facilities	Importance of HMO patients to practice
Staff Model	Salary	HMO	Only patients
Group Model	Fixed capitation, profit sharing	HMO	Core
Network Model	Negotiated capitation	Practice	Less important
Individual Practice Association (IPA)	Many contracts, negotiated fee schedules	Practice	Secondary

Preferred provider organization (PPO) is fee-for-service at a discount. In a PPO, the insurance company contracts to provide services at a present price or discount. The discount is substantial: often 30% below standard fees for primary care and 50% below standard fees for specialists. In exchange for discount, insurer agrees to provide incentives for patient to use contracted providers.

Provider makes money on volume, i.e., less money per patient but more patients. Efficiency is rewarded. Provider is limited in ability to raise prices. Insurance company conducts utilization review to be sure that only appropriate services are delivered and billed. Providers may "bid for patients," seeking greater volume by offering deeper discounts.

GOVERNMENT METHODS OF PAYMENT FOR SERVICES

Medicare: Federal government program that makes health care payments to those on Social Security. Program pays health care costs for the elderly (age >65), disabled, and dependents of disabled. Part A pays for hospital care; part B pays for physician services. Annual deductibles and copayments are applicable. Patient can use up Medicare benefits. If providers accept "assignment," they must accept Medicare-set fees only.

Covered services include: hospital stays; laboratory workups; non-self-administered drugs; ambulatory surgery; physical, speech, and occupational therapy; rehabilitation; kidney dialysis; ambulance transport; diabetes testing equipment; pneumococcal and hepatitis B vaccination. Some prescription coverage is available for an added fee. Services *not* covered: routine physicals; eye/ear examinations for glasses/hearing aids; immunizations; routine foot care; custodial (nursing home) care; most self-administered drugs.

Medicaid: health care payments for those on welfare. A joint state/federal program that covers all care, including hospital stays, physician services, medication, and nursing homes. However, Medicaid payments to providers are generally far below standard fees. If poor and over age 65, Medicare is first used, then Medicaid. No deductibles, copayments, or fees. Each state sets eligibility, services covered, and administration, hence wide differences across the United States.

Diagnostic-related groups (DRGs) are payment categories used to classify patients (especially Medicare patients) for the purpose of reimbursing hospitals for each case in a given category, There is a fixed fee, regardless of the actual costs incurred, since patients within each category are clinically similar and are expected to use the same level of hospital resources. DRGs have been used in the United States since the early 1980s to determine how much Medicare pays the hospital for services. They are assigned based on diagnosis, procedure, age, sex, discharge status, and presence of complications or comorbidities.

DRGs limit what the government will pay (but does not set prices). Prospective payment is set by taking national median cost to treat each of approximately 500 different diagnoses. Payment is determined by adding or subtracting from this median cost according to a formula that includes principal and up to 4 secondary diagnoses, principal procedures, patient's age, patient's gender, patient's discharge status, prevailing wage rate in the area, extra payments for teaching hospitals, and extra payments also for "outliers": patients costing far beyond usual expenses.

Consequences of DRGs include more outpatient treatment, quicker discharges from hospital, serial admissions (new payments after 31 days), inflation in number of diagnoses, preferences for certain diagnoses and procedures that pay more, upcoding (recording a diagnosis that pays more, which is illegal).

DRGs generally do not apply to psychiatric, pediatric, or physical rehabilitation cases.

Resource-based relative-value scale (RBRVS) is a program used to determine how much money providers should be compensated. It is used by Medicare and HMOs. This program assigns a relative value to procedures and services performed, and is adjusted by geographic region. Sets government payments to physicians (and insurance companies, as well). Pays fairly well, but takes capacity to set fees away from individual providers. Payments are made using a formula that includes amount of time, work, skill, and effort required; typical costs of physician's practice (including malpractice premiums); typical cost of physician's postgraduate (residency, fellowship) training; typical office overhead.

Consequences of RBRVS are higher payments to primary care, lower payments to procedure-based specialties, and higher payments for cognitive work (talking with and thinking about the patient).

SECTION III

Social Sciences

Basic Science of Patient Safety 16

Learning Objectives

- ❏ Answer questions about scope of patient safety problems
- ❏ Describe the categories of medical error
- ❏ Answer questions about the systems approach to medical error and failure analysis
- ❏ Analyze cases concerning error disclosure and reporting
- ❏ Demonstrate understanding of principles of quality improvement
- ❏ Explain the leadership role of physician to lead change in patient safety

INTRODUCTION

Case 1: Care done well

A 3-year-old girl falls into an icy fishpond in a small Austrian town in the Alps. She is lost beneath the surface for 30 minutes before her parents find her on the pond bottom and pull her up. CPR is started immediately by the parents on instruction from an emergency physician on the phone, and EMS arrives within 8 minutes. The girl has a body temperature of 19° C and no pulse. Her pupils are dilated and do not react to light. A helicopter takes the patient to a nearby hospital where she is wheeled directly to an operating room. A surgical team puts her on a heart-lung bypass machine, her body temperature increases nearly 10 degrees, and her heart begins to beat. She requires placement on extracorporeal membrane oxygenation. Over the next few days her body temperature continues to rise to normal, and the organs start to recover. She suffered extensive neurologic deficits; however, by age 5, after extensive outpatient therapy, she recovers completely and is like any other little girl again.

Case 2: Failure of the medical system

A newborn baby boy is first noted to be jaundiced through visual assessment hours after delivery, but a bilirubin test is not done. At the time of discharge from the hospital, the child is described as having 'head to toe jaundice,' but a bilirubin test had still not been done, nor had his blood type or Coombs test been performed. The parents are instructed that the jaundice is normal and they should not worry, and to simply place the infant in the window for sunlight. A few days later the baby's mother calls the newborn nursery stating that her son is still yellow, lethargic, and feeding poorly. She is asked if she is a "first-time mom" and then assured that there was no concern. The mother continues to notice that the child is not well. At age 5 days, the mother's concerns are acknowledged and a pediatrician admits the baby boy to the pediatric unit. On day 6 in the afternoon, the child has a high pitched cry, respiratory distress, and increased tone. He also starts to arch his neck in a way that is characteristic of opisthotonos. The child is ultimately diagnosed with classic textbook kernicterus, resulting in permanent brain damage.

The 2 real cases above represent the reality of our current health care system and the issues of patient safety. In one case a series of complex processes result in an excellent outcome, while in another a patient suffers preventable injury.

What are the factors that cause a good versus poor outcome? The field of patient safety seeks to answer this question and take steps to prevent future patients from being harmed by medical errors.

Patients are at risk for sustaining harm from the health care system and do so at an alarmingly high rate. Injury can range from minor to severe incidents, including death. The cause of these adverse events is not usually intentional injury (i.e. someone intending to harm patients), but rather is due to the complexity of the health care system combined with the inherent capability of human error.

The prevalence of medical errors in the United States is a significant and ongoing problem. Media reports of catastrophic injury resulting in disability or death due to medical care often reach news headlines, and are a significant concern to patients, families, and members of the health care team. The causes of these errors are varied, and can include failures in the administration of medication, performing surgery, reporting laboratory results, and diagnosing patients, to name a few.

Ensuring patient safety is the responsibility of every member of the health care team. To do so requires an understanding of safety science and quality improvement principles. Patients, providers, payers, and employers are all stakeholders in improving patient safety. Applying these principles to the study of medical errors can help health care professionals learn from past errors and develop systems that prevent future errors from harming subsequent patients. Systems in health care delivery can be redesigned to create safeguards and safety nets which make it difficult for members of the health care team to make errors that harm patients. The goal of health care should be to learn the strategies and systems that are currently being put into place to improve patient safety.

SCOPE OF THE PROBLEM

In 1999 the Institute of Medicine (IOM) published its landmark publication, 'To Err is Human: Building a Safer Health System,' reporting that at least 44,000 people—and perhaps as many as 98,000—die in hospitals each year as a result of medical errors that could have been prevented. This exceeds deaths attributed to breast cancer, motor vehicle collisions, and HIV. Approximately 1 in 10 patients entering the hospital will suffer harm from an adverse event.

Patient harm from preventable medical errors is a serious concern in health care. The impact of these errors can have dramatically negative effects on patients, their families, and the health care personnel involved. In addition to the toll on human suffering, medical errors also present a significant source of inefficiency and increased cost in the health care system.

Medical errors are the eighth leading cause of wrongful death in the United States. The problem is not limited to this country, however; medical errors are a global problem.

Some of the more common contributors to medical errors and adverse patient events are as follows:

Medication errors represent one of the most common causes of preventable patient harm. An estimated 1.5 million deaths occur each year in the United States due to medication error. The IOM estimates that 1 medication error occurs per hospitalized patient each day.

Common causes of medication error:

- Poor handwriting technique on a prescription pad or order form, resulting in a pharmacist or nurse administering the wrong drug or wrong dose
- Dosing or route of administration errors
- Failure to identify that given patient is allergic to a prescribed medication
- Look-alike or sound-alike drugs (e.g., rifampin/rifiximin)

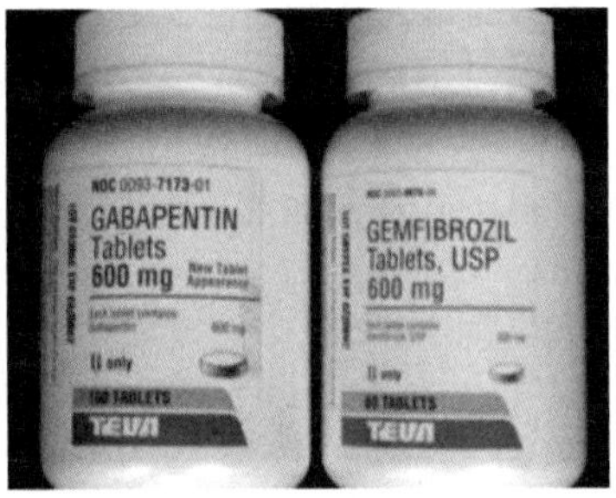

Figure 16-1. 'Look-Alike' Medications

Strategies that help to reduce or prevent medication errors are as follows.

- The **5 Rs** help to confirm several key points before the administration of any medication.
  - Right drug
  - Right patient
  - Right dose
  - Right route
  - Right time
- Computerized physician order entry (CPOE) involves entering medication orders directly into a computer system rather than on paper or verbally. The computer software (i.e. electronic health record) can automatically check for prescribing errors or allergies.

Hospital-acquired infections (HAI) affect 5-15% of all hospitalized patients and 40% of patients in ICU. The World Health Organization (WHO) estimates that the mortality from health-care-associated infections ranges from 12–80%.

HAI can occur in many forms, the most common of which in hospitalized patients is **urinary catheter-related infection** (UTI). UTI accounts for 40% of all HAI; >80% of these infections are attributable to use of an indwelling urethral catheter. Adhering to strict indications for using indwelling catheters, maintaining sterile technique during catheter insertion and exercising prompt removal of the catheter when it is no longer required can help reduce the risk of a urinary catheter-related infection.

Central line associated bloodstream infection (CLABSI) is another common HAI, and among one of the most common infections observed in patients admitted to critical care units. It is estimated that 70% of hospital-acquired bloodstream infections occur in patients with central venous catheters. Symptoms include fever, chills, erythema at the skin surrounding the central line site and, in severe cases, hypotension secondary to sepsis. These infections can be associated with significant morbidity and mortality, increased length of hospital stay, and increased hospital cost. Checklists have been developed which provide best practices for the placement of central lines that lower the risk of infection (e.g., hand washing, gloving and gowning, sterile barriers, and early removal of central lines when possible).

Hospital-acquired pneumonia (HAP) is an infection that occurs more often in ventilated patients, typically $\geq$48 hours after admission to a hospital. These ventilator-associated pneumonias (VAP), a subtype of HAP, tend to be more serious because patients are often sicker and less able to mount effective immune responses. HAP is the second most common nosocomial infection. Common symptoms include coughing, fever, chills, fatigue, malaise, headache, loss of appetite, nausea and vomiting, shortness of breath, and sharp or stabbing chest pain that gets worse with deep breathing or coughing. Several methods have been undertaken to prevent HAP, including infection control (e.g. hand hygiene and proper use of gloves, gown and mask), elevation of the head of the bed in ventilated patients, and other measures to reduce the risk of aspiration.

Surgical site infections (SSI) occur following a surgical procedure in the part of the body where the surgery took place. Some SSIs are superficial and limited to the skin, while others are more serious and involve deep tissue under the skin, body cavities, internal organs, or implanted material (e.g. knee or hip replacements). Symptoms include fever, drainage of cloudy fluid from the surgical incision or erythema and tenderness at the surgical site. Most superficial SSIs (e.g., cellulitis) can be treated with appropriate antibiotics, whereas deeper infections (i.e., abscess) require drainage. Pre-operative antibiotics have been effective in reducing the rate of SSIs.

Patient falls are a common cause of injury in hospitals and other health care settings such as nursing homes. Over $\frac{1}{3}$ of elderly people age >65 fall each year. Researchers estimate that >500,000 falls happen each year in U.S. hospitals, resulting in 150,000 injuries. Approximately 30% of inpatient falls result in injury, with 4–6% resulting in serious injury. Injuries can include bone fractures, head injury, bleeding, and even death. Injuries from falls also increase hospital costs.

Assessing a patient's fall risk helps to identify high-risk patients who can benefit from preventative resources. Some risk factors include advanced age (age >60), muscle weakness, taking >4 prescription medications (especially sedatives, hypnotics, antidepressants, or benzodiazepines), impaired memory, and difficulty walking (e.g. use of a cane or walker). Interventions such as increased observation, nonslip footwear, and making the environment safe all play a role in preventing injury from falls.

Unplanned readmissions occur when patients unexpectantly return to the hospital <30 days after being discharged. According to a *New England Journal of Medicine* study analyzing close to 12 million Medicare beneficiaries, nearly 20% of those discharged were readmitted within 30 days. Several factors can lead to a hospital readmission, such as poor quality of care or breakdowns in communication during a transition of care (e.g. hospital to rehabilitation center). Readmissions may also occur if patients are discharged from hospitals prematurely, are discharged to inappropriate settings, or if they do not receive adequate information or resources to aid in recovery.

For example, a 79-year-old patient treated for congestive heart failure (CHF) returns to the hospital 10 days after discharge with exacerbation of CHF. It was discovered that upon release the patient had failed to fill the prescription for the diuretic started during the initial hospitalization. Improving communication, patient education and providing appropriate support to patients at risk for readmissions are all strategies to reduce unplanned readmissions.

CAUSES OF MEDICAL ERROR

The miraculous recovery of the little girl after the drowning event in case 1 highlights the incredible complexity of our modern health delivery system. There were numerous steps that were required to get right in the care of the patient. Unfortunately, these steps are not always followed as well as they were in that case. Machines break down, a team can't get moving fast enough, or a simple step is forgotten or the wrong step applied. The greater the number of steps required, the greater the risk of something going wrong. Couple that with the fact that human beings are prone to error, especially when working under less-than-ideal circumstances, and it is no wonder that medical errors pose such a threat to health care.

The complexity of the health care system, together with the potential for mistakes due to human nature, is the primary reason that patients experience medical errors. Understanding medical error and the science of patient safety can help us design a health care system capable of getting it right every time.

The potential for human error is amplified by poor working conditions. This includes poor workplace conditions (e.g., overworked staff, time pressures, lack of safety protocols or lack of appropriate supervision), as well as poor individual conditions (e.g., fatigue, stress or illness).

Note

Errors are bound to occur due to a combination of a complex health care system and the reality of human fallibility.

The following is a mnemonic to help assess the fitness of a health care professional to attend to patient care.

IM SAFE

I: Illness (Are you suffering from an illness that is degrading your performance?)

M: Medications (Are you taking medications that may impair your judgment?)

S: Stress (Are you adequately managing the stressors in your life?)

A: Alcohol (Are you using alcohol in excess with negative consequences?)

F: Fatigue (Are you getting enough rest?)

E: Eating (Are you maintaining a healthy diet?)

For example, one study on physician performance found that being awake 24 hours was equivalent to having a blood alcohol level of .10 (legally intoxicated by most standards) (Dawson & Reid, 1997).

Communication and teamwork failures are another leading cause of adverse patient events. Lack of appropriate communication creates situations where medical errors are likely to occur. These errors have the potential to cause severe injury and unexpected patient death. Errors at the time of transitions or handoffs are among the most common communication errors in healthcare. Handoffs occur frequently between nurses and between residents in teaching hospitals, but also among attending faculty (e.g., on-call physicians, hospitalists, ED staff). Using techniques of structured communication (e.g., SBAR, call-backs) can help safeguard against errors. Poor teamwork and lack of coordination between members of the patient care team also result in medical errors. A growing recognition of the need for improved teamwork in health care has led to the application of teamwork training principles, originally developed in aviation, to a variety of clinical settings. Recognized barriers to effective teamwork include:

- Inconsistency in team membership
- Lack of time
- Lack of Information Sharing
- Hierarchy
- Defensiveness
- Conventional Thinking
- Complacency
- Varying Communication Styles
- Conflict
- Lack of Coordination
- Distractions
- Fatigue
- Workload
- Misinterpretation of Cues
- Lack of Role Clarity

Teamwork training attempts to reduce the potential for patient harm by developing effective communication skills, a supportive working environment, and an atmosphere in which all team members feel comfortable speaking up when they suspect a problem. Team members are trained to cross-monitor; check each other's actions, offer assistance when needed, and address errors in a nonjudgmental fashion (i.e. watch each other's backs). Huddles, Briefs and Debriefs are essential components of teamwork training; as is providing feedback, especially after critical incidents. Remember, a chain is only as strong as its weakest link.

TYPES OF MEDICAL ERROR

Types of Errors

Diagnostic

- Error or delay in diagnosis
- Failure to employ indicated tests
- Use of outmoded tests or therapy
- Failure to act on results of monitoring or testing

Treatment

- Error in the performance of an operation, procedure, or test
- Error in administering the treatment
- Error in the dose or method of using a drug
- Avoidable delay in treatment or in responding to an abnormal test inappropriate (not indicated) care

Preventive

- Failure to provide prophylactic treatment
- Inadequate monitoring or follow-up of treatment
- Other
  - Failure of communication
  - Equipment failure
  - Other system failure

Source: Leape, Lucian; Lawthers, Ann G.; Brennan, Troyen A., et al. Preventing Medical Injury. Qual Rev Bull. 19(5): 144–149, 1993

Errors can be categorized as slips, lapses, or mistakes.

- **Slips** can be thought of as actions not carried out as intended or planned e.g. injecting a medication intravenously when you meant to give it subcutaneously. Slips are observable.
- **Lapses** are missed actions and omissions (e.g. forgetting to monitor and replace serum potassium in a patient treated with furosemide for acute congestive heart failure). Lapses are generally not observable (i.e. one cannot directly 'see' a lapse of memory).

Both slips and lapses are actions that do not 'go as intended.'

- **Mistakes** are a specific type of error brought about by a faulty plan or incorrect intentions; the intended action is wrong (e.g. extubating a patient prematurely based on misapplication of guidelines, or treating a patient for a suspected pneumonia when the patient was misdiagnosed and actually has a pulmonary embolism).

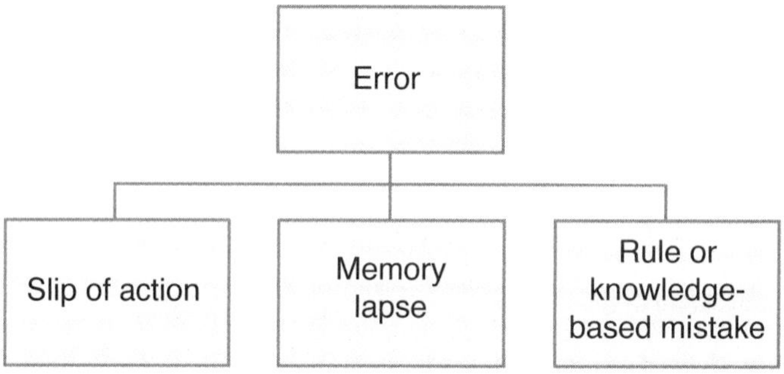

Figure 16-2. Types of Error

It is important to differentiate errors (slip, lapse, or mistake) from violations.

- **Violations** are deliberate actions, whereby someone does something and knows it to be against the rules (e.g. deliberately failing to follow proper procedures). A health care professional may consider that a violation is well-intentioned; however, it would still technically constitute a 'violation' rather than an error. For example, a physician may decide to forgo entering a patient's allergies into the electronic record due to time constraints in starting treatment. If this act led to an adverse medication reaction due to a missed allergic reaction, it would technically be considered a violation and not an error.

Errors may result in adverse events or near-misses.

- **Adverse events** are harms or injuries that result directly from medical care, not from negative outcomes due to the patient's disease or medical condition.
- **Near-misses** are errors that occur but do not result in injury or harm to patients because they are caught in time or simply because of luck.

Diagnostic errors account for at least 17% of preventable errors in hospitalized patients. Diagnostic errors can be categorized as no-fault, system-related, and cognitive.

- **No-fault errors** may happen when there are masked or unusual symptoms of a disease, or when a patient has not fully cooperated in care.
- **System-related** errors include technical failure, equipment problems and organizational flaws.
- **Cognitive errors** frequently result from a diagnosis that was wrong, missed, or unintentionally delayed due to clinician error.

The following are examples of common cognitive errors.

A wrong diagnosis may occur when the clinician holds on to a particular diagnosis (usually the initial one, in a phenomenon called **anchoring bias**) and becomes dismissive to signs and symptoms pointing to another diagnosis. For example, a 65-year-old man presents with epigastric pain, and emesis, and he sits leaning forward. He has a history of alcoholism. The patient is likely to be diagnosed with pancreatitis. However, holding on to this diagnosis to the exclusion of any other diagnosis—despite the patient's denial of alcohol use for several years, normal blood levels of pancreatic enzymes, and abnormal EKG which is ignored—would be an anchoring error.

Confirmation bias, looking for evidence to support a pre-conceived opinion, rather than looking for evidence that refutes it or provides greater support to an alternative diagnosis, may accompany an anchoring error. Clinicians should regard conflicting data as evidence for the need to continue to seek the true diagnosis (e.g. in the case above; acute MI) rather than as anomalies to be disregarded.

Availability bias is the tendency to assume a diagnosis based on recent patient encounters or memorable cases (i.e., the most cognitively "available" diagnosis).

It is estimated that thousands of hospitalized patients die every year due to diagnostic errors. Missed or delayed diagnoses (particularly of cancer) are a prominent reason for malpractice claims. Poor teamwork/communication between clinicians and a lack of reliable systems for common outpatient clinical situations (e.g., triaging acutely ill patients by telephone and following-up on test results) have been identified as predisposing factors for diagnostic error.

SYSTEMS APPROACH TO MEDICAL ERROR

Health professionals dedicate their lives to the care of patients. Most are highly trained and competent; however, the nature of health care is extremely complex, and people, despite good intentions, are still capable of making errors.

Although hospitals, clinics, and doctor's offices take many steps to keep their patients safe, medical errors can, and do, occur. Rather than penalize individuals who make honest mistakes, the goal of patient safety is to redesign systems to be more fool-proof and able to compensate for human error.

Bad Apples/Blame Culture: When a medical error occurs, the bad apple approach seeks to identify who is responsible for the error and take punitive action against that individual. However, this approach does not improve safety. It creates a culture of fear and doesn't address the root cause of the error.

Only 5% of patient harm is due directly to incompetence or poor intentions. People need to be accountable, but systems changes are needed to truly transform care. Unfortunately, health care has a long tradition of a blame culture. Blaming people who make errors does not get to underlying causes or help to prevent the error from happening to someone else in the future.

The most effective approach to reducing harm from medical error is to find out *how* the error happened, rather than who did it, and then fix the system to prevent errors from causing injury to patients. Improvements in patient safety will be hindered as long as there is a focus on blaming individuals.

SYSTEMS APPROACH TO FAILURE

An understanding of medical error requires an understanding of the systems failures underlying the majority of adverse patient events. Health care is a complex system. Errors that harm patients tend to have multiple causes that are ingrained in this complex system. James Reason, a pioneer and leader in the research area of human error and organizational processes, describes the **Swiss Cheese Model** of accident causation; it is a model used in risk analysis and risk management in complex systems including health care.

The Swiss cheese model encompasses the understanding that patient harm often results from multiple, upstream or proximal errors. In the Swiss cheese model, each 'slice' represents a barrier, and each hole is a failure in the system due to either active or latent failures. Under normal circumstances one of the barriers works to prevent patient harm (e.g. the nurse catches that the medication ordered is the wrong dose before giving it to the patient); however, occasionally the perfect storm scenario arises where the holes line up and allow an error to reach the patient resulting in harm.

For example, if the hazard were wrong-site orthopedic surgery, slices of cheese might include policies for identifying sidedness on radiology imaging, a protocol for signing the correct site when the surgeon and patient meet in the preoperative area, and a second protocol for reviewing the medical record and checking the previously marked site in the operating room. Many more layers exist but the point is that no single barrier is foolproof. They each have "holes," hence, the Swiss cheese.

Note

Approximately 80% of medical errors or adverse patient events are system-derived.

In some serious events such as wrong site surgery, even though the holes will only align infrequently, the result is still unacceptable patient injury. For instance, in an emergency situation, all 3 of the surgical identification safety checks mentioned above may fail or be bypassed, resulting in the surgeon meeting the patient for the first time in the operating room already under anesthesia. A hurried x-ray technologist might mislabel a film (or simply hang it backward and a hurried surgeon may not notice), confirming the surgical site with the patient may not take place at all (e.g. if the patient is unconscious) or, if it takes place, be rushed and offer no real protection.

Under the blame culture traditionally present in health care, a person may be reprimanded for an error but the holes in the system are not addressed; making it quite probable that the same error will be committed by someone else in the future leading to more patient harm. The goal is to examine the system and develop methods to redesign care so that the holes are removed.

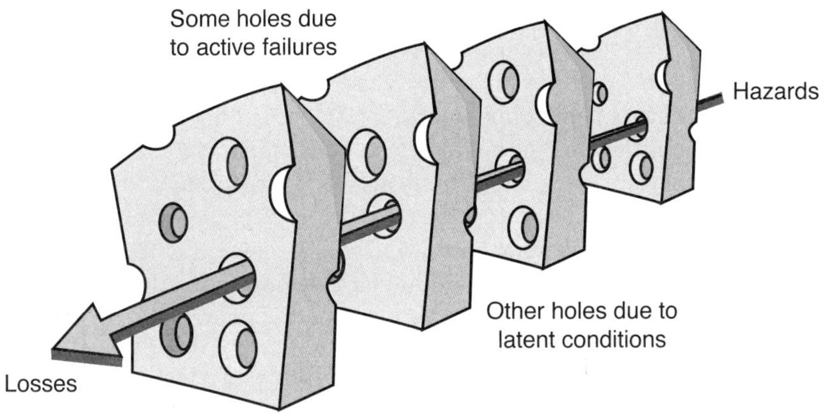

Source: James Reason

Figure 16-3. Successive Layers of Defenses, Barriers, and Safeguards

Other industries with complex systems, such as aviation and nuclear power plants, have successfully employed systems engineering to drastically improve safety and reliability. These industries have also made changes to improve communication, teamwork, and the culture of safety.

Another example of lessons learned from systems engineering is the automobile safety industry. Most motor vehicle collision (MVC) deaths are due to driver error or deliberate misbehavior (e.g. speeding, running a red light, failure to wear a seatbelt, etc.). The death toll from MVC in the past several decades has declined significantly. Drivers today are not necessarily safer drivers than before; however, design changes in cars (e.g. collapsible steering columns, airbags) and safe highway design (e.g. improved lighting, deformable lampposts) have resulted in drastic reductions in mortality from MVCs.

Likewise, the goal in patient safety is to prevent errors from resulting in harm to patients. Health care must create safety nets that absorb mistakes before they reach patients. Some examples of system-based redesigns for patient safety include protocols to ensure proper patient identification, such as the following:

- Using at least 2 methods such as patient name and date of birth to confirm patient identify prior to the administration of medications
- Using a standardized pre-operative checklist to help operating room staff review critical information prior to surgery (e.g. pre-operative antibiotics)
- Removing look-alike drugs from the nursing unit in order to prevent medication errors

ERROR DISCLOSURE AND REPORTING

Many victims of medical errors never learn that the mistake occurred, because the error is simply not disclosed. Healthcare professionals have traditionally shied away from discussing errors with patients, due to fear of precipitating a malpractice lawsuit, issues of professional embarrassment or discomfort with the disclosure process. It is both an ethical and professional responsibility to ensure that errors resulting in patient harm are disclosed and reported.

The first priority after an event which causes patient harm is to care for the patient's medical needs. **Disclosure** of the error is another important early action. Following an adverse event, patients and families want to hear an apology and to know what is being done to prevent the error from harming someone else in the future. They may also require emotional and social support. Honesty and transparency are essential. There is no role for covering up an error (e.g. altering documentation to conceal the error) or withholding information from the patient or family. Such practices are unethical and betray the professional responsibility we have to patients. Studies have demonstrated that a timely and sincere apology may actually reduce the likelihood of a lawsuit.

Often the most senior physician responsible for the patient and most familiar with the case will make the official disclosure. An error disclosure should include the following 3 elements:

- Accurate description of the events and their impact on the patient
- Sincere apology showing care and compassion
- Assurance that appropriate steps are being taken to prevent the adverse event from happening to another patient in the future

Reporting allows for errors to be studied so that system-based improvements can be made to help prevent such errors from harming patients in the future. Reporting errors is essential for error prevention and provides opportunities to improve processes of care by learning from failures of the health care system. In order to be effective, reporting must be safe. Individuals who report incidents must not be punished or suffer other ill-effects from reporting. The fear of punitive retaliation or other negative consequences will serve as an impediment to incident reporting. The identities of reporters should not normally be disclosed to third parties.

Other barriers to error reporting include the belief that that no corrective action will be taken and having an overly burdensome reporting system. To overcome these barriers, reported events should be reviewed and acted upon in a timely fashion, and the system for reporting errors should be made as straightforward as possible.

One other recognized barrier to error reporting is failure to recognize that an error has occurred. For example, an interventional cardiologist accidentally orders the wrong dose of medication during a cardiac catheterization; however, the nurse who has worked with this cardiologist for years knows the correct dose intended and makes the appropriate adjustment. No harm has occurred but it would be wrong not to realize that an error did happen.

Health care professionals need to be educated about medical error identification, including the identification and importance of near-misses. Although near-misses (errors that occur but fortunately do not result in patient harm) do not generally need to be disclosed to patients, they should still be reported to the system so that they, too, can be studied. One person's near-miss may be the next person's fatal error. Estimates of the scope of medical errors likely do not reflect the numerous near-misses that do not result in patient harm.

Note

Estimates are that voluntarily reported medical errors only reflect 10–20% of actual errors.

It is important to have a culture that promotes error reporting and error analysis in order to enhance health systems. Every error represents an opportunity to improve a process; however, in order to improve, these errors must be recognized and made known so that system-wide learning and performance can take place.

ANALYSIS OF MEDICAL ERRORS

A systematic approach for understanding the cause of adverse events and identifying flaws in the system which can be corrected to prevent harm in the future is called **root cause analysis** (RCA). RCA is *retrospective* in nature; the focus is on systems and process rather than individual blame. The question asked is, "**how did this happen?**," not "whose fault is this?" The goal is to determine why an event happened and what can be done to prevent it from happening again. RCA is not applicable to negligence or willful harm.

A classic tool used in RCA is the **Fishbone** or **Ishikawa diagram** (also known as a **Cause and Effect diagram**), which analyzes a complex system and identifies possible causes for an effect or problem. This type of diagram is used to explore and display all the possible causes of a particular error.

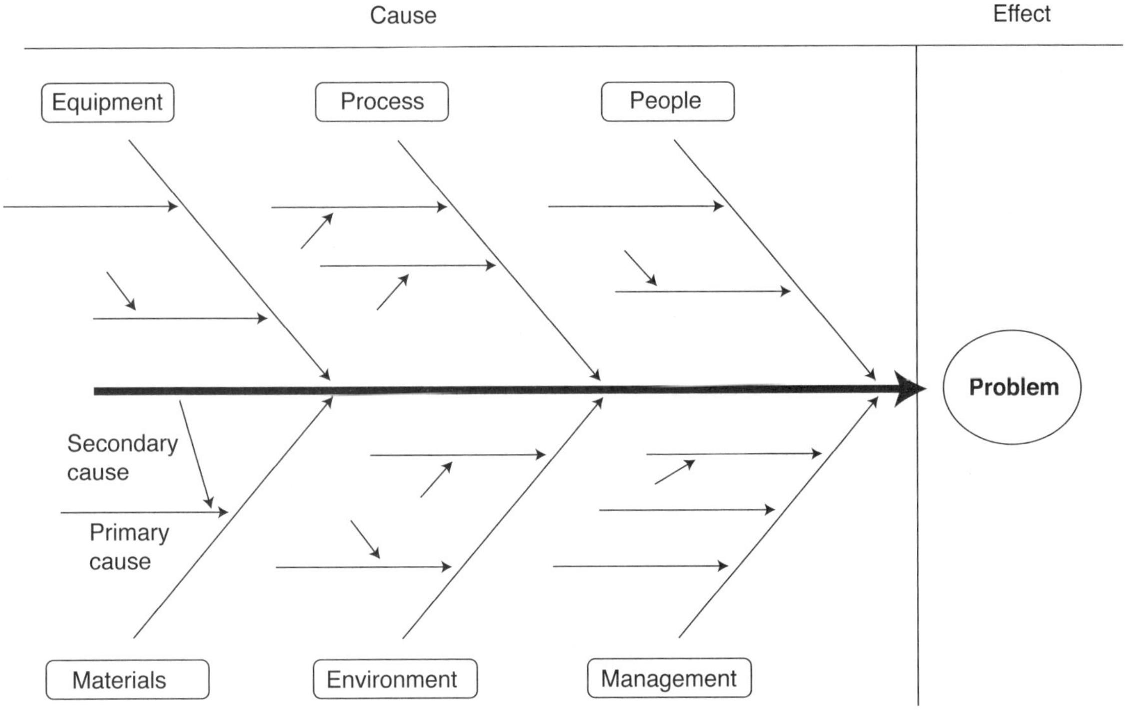

Figure 16-4. Sample Fishbone (Ishikawa) Diagram

The RCA allows the team to identify problems in the system or process of care. The end product of the RCA process is a list of recommended actions to prevent the recurrence of the adverse event in the future. Recommendations commonly consist of one or more of the following actions: standardizing equipment, using double checks or backup systems, employing forcing functions that physically prevent users from making common mistakes, making changes to the physical set-up, updating or improving technology, using cognitive aids (e.g. checklists or mnemonic devices), simplifying a process, educating staff or implementing new safety policies.

In contrast to the retrospective nature of RCA, the prospective failure mode effects analysis (FMEA) is an engineering approach which seeks to anticipate and prevent adverse events through safety design. The goal of FMEA is to prevent patient problems before they occur. FMEA is a systematic and proactive approach that seeks to identify possible failures in the system and potential weaknesses in order to develop strategies to prevent the failures from occurring.

PRINCIPLES OF QUALITY IMPROVEMENT

> 'Every system is perfectly designed to get the results it gets.'
>
> \- Source: Don Berwick, M.D.

A key principle of quality improvement is to design systems capable of identifying, preventing, absorbing and mitigating errors. Some everyday examples of safety design outside of health care are seatbelt alarms in cars, heat-sensitive fire sprinkler systems, and tip-over switches which automatically turn off space heaters that have accidentally fallen over.

In 2001, the IOM published a report, "Crossing the Quality Chasm" which aimed at promoting fundamental changes in health care in order to close the quality gap. The report recommended a redesign of the American health care system and provided principles for guiding quality improvement. Specifically, the report defined 6 aims of health care (STEEEP):

1. **Safe**: avoidance of injuries to patients from the care that is intended to help them
2. **Timely**: reduce waits and harmful delays in care
3. **Effective**: provide care based on scientific knowledge likely to benefit patients
4. **Efficient**: avoid waste in equipment, supplies, ideas, and energy
5. **Equitable**: provide care that does not vary in quality because of personal characteristics such as gender, ethnicity, geographic location, and socioeconomic status
6. **Patient-centered**: provide care that is respectful of and responsive to individual patient preferences, needs, and values

Another significant initiative in quality improvement is the Institute for Health Care Improvements (IHI) Triple Aim that describes an approach to optimizing health system performance using new designs to pursue 3 dimensions (i.e. "Triple Aim").

- Improve the patient experience of care (including quality and satisfaction)
- Improve the health of populations
- Reduce per capita cost of health care

Measures of Quality

There are 3 traditional categories of measures used in quality improvement: structure, process, and outcomes.

- **Structure** relates to the physical equipment, resources, or facilities (e.g., number of ICU beds in a hospital).
- **Process** relates to how the system works (e.g. how often nurses use bar coding to identify patients prior to administering medication).
- **Outcomes** represent the final product or end result in patient care (e.g. infection rate in pediatric hematology patients admitted to the hospital). Outcomes are often difficult to assess in quality improvement, and many people often use process measures as a surrogate for outcomes. For example, it may be difficult to accurately track all HAI (*outcomes measure*), so rates of compliance with hand washing are monitored instead (*process measure*).

A fourth type of measure introduced to quality improvement is the concept of a balancing measure. **Balancing measures** ask whether changes made to improve one part of the system cause an unanticipated decrease in performance in another part of the system (e.g. did an initiative aimed at increasing the efficiency of discharging patients from the hospital lead to more patients being sent home without appropriate follow-up instructions).

Models of Quality Improvement

One example of a common quality improvement model is a combination of building and applying knowledge to make an improvement by asking 3 questions and using the **PDSA** (plan, do, study, act) cycle developed by W. Edwards Deming, a pioneer and influential leader in quality control.

1. What are we trying to accomplish?
2. How will we know whether a change is an improvement?
3. What changes can we make that will result in an improvement?

This model takes the simple concept of "trial and error" and transforms it into the PDSA model that can be used to make improvements in health care.

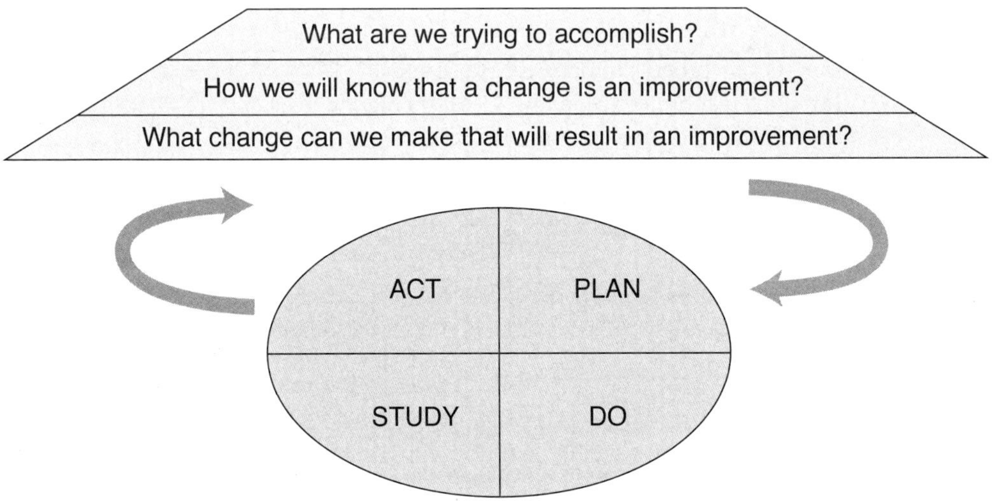

Source: Langley, Nolan, Nolan & Provost 1999

Figure 16-5. The Model for Improvement

- **Plan**: plan a change or a pilot test of a new intervention or innovation
- **Do**: carry out the plan
- **Study**: evaluate the results
- **Act**: decide what actions should be taken to improve (i.e. implement the new intervention or start over with a new plan based on the prior results)

Six Sigma is another model for quality improvement with origins from the manufacturing industry. The term comes from the use in statistics of the Greek Letter (sigma) to denote Standard Deviation from the mean. Six sigma is equivalent to 3.4 defects (or errors) per million. This system uses specific steps to reduce variation and improve performance.

- DMAIC (define – measure – analyze – improve - control): an improvement system for **existing processes** falling below specification
  - **Define**: Define the problem in detail.
  - **Measure**: Measure defects (in terms of "defects per million," or Sigma level).
  - **Analyze**: Do in-depth analysis using process measures, flow charts and defect analysis to determine the conditions under which defects occur.
  - **Improve**: Define and test changes aimed at reducing defects.
  - **Control**: What steps will you take to maintain performance?

Lean (also called Lean Enterprise or Toyota Production System) is an improvement process that seeks to improve value from the patient's perspective, by reducing waste in time and resources that do not enhance patient outcomes. This includes certain lab tests, imaging studies or care services that may be commonly performed, but in reality do not actually help the patient. For example, a pre-operative EKG obtained on a healthy 21 year-old with no cardiac symptoms undergoing a small outpatient procedure can be considered a wasteful test that does not help the patient.

Flowcharts allow health care teams to understand the steps involved in the delivery of patient care service. A flowchart is a visual illustration of all the steps or parts of a process in patient care. There are 2 types of flowcharts: **high-level flowcharts** (more conceptually focused, 'big picture') and **detailed flowcharts** (more focused on specific, fine points).

Flowcharts are more accurate and effective when all representative members of a health care team actively participate in their design. They help health-care providers achieve a shared understanding of a clinical process and use that knowledge as the basis for designing new ways to improve services. Specifically, they can help to identify steps that do not add value to the process (e.g. unnecessary duplication of services), to determine areas of delay in care, and to discover failure points in the system.

Pareto charts are used to describe a large proportion of quality problems being caused by a small number of causes. It is based on the classic $\frac{80}{20}$ rule from economics, where 80% of the world's wealth is described to be in the hands of an elite 20% of the population.

The Pareto principle applied to health care states that the **majority of patient safety errors stem from only a few recurring contributing factors**, which should serve as the focus the problem-solving efforts. In essence, it is a method of prioritizing problems, highlighting the fact that most problems are affected by a few factors and indicating which problems to solve and in what order. A Pareto chart includes the multiple factors that contribute to an effect arranged in descending order (according to the magnitude of their effect). The ordering is an important step because it helps the team concentrate efforts on those factors that have the greatest impact

Run charts (or time plots) are graphs of data collected over time which can help determine whether an intervention or enhancement in the patient care process has resulted in true improvement over time or rather if it simply represents a random fluctuation (that might be incorrectly interpreted as a significant improvement). Run charts are created by plotting time along the X-axis (e.g. minutes, hours, days, months) and the quality measure on the Y-axis (e.g. number of infections, wait times, falls). The median (or 50th percentile) is measured using baseline historical data and then compared to outcomes measured following the quality improvement intervention.

Run charts help identify whether there is a true trend vs. a random-pattern. A shift in the process signaling a significant change in quality can be identified, for example, by observing ≥6 consecutive points above or below the median, or by ≥5 consecutive points all increasing or decreasing.

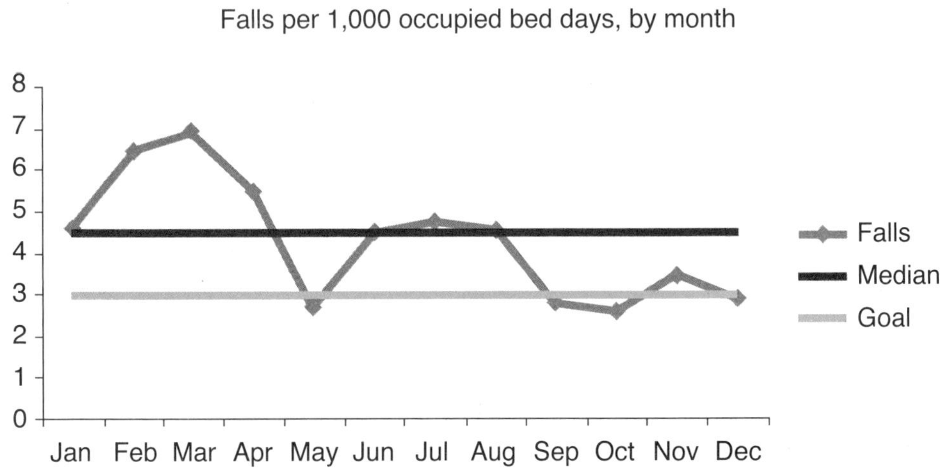

Figure 16-6. Sample Run Chart Plotting Patient Falls (ahrq.gov)

A Shewhart (or control chart) applies formal statistical calculations (statistical process control) to determine whether the observed rise and fall of a quality measure over time is within a predictable range of variation or is an indication of a significant change in the system. Control charts use upper and lower control limits (sometimes called "natural process limits") which indicate the threshold at which the process output is considered statistically 'unlikely,' and are drawn typically at 3 standard errors from the center line.

A **convenience sample** is the study group or population used in the test of a quality improvement initiative. Using convenience sampling is an efficient and simple method to test an intervention. This is not the same process often used in randomized controlled trials, and thus may not be an accurate reflection of the larger group. Ideally, however, the sample will have approximately similar characteristics to the larger population.

LEADING CHANGE IN PATIENT SAFETY

Patient safety is the professional responsibility of everyone on the patient care team. In order to effect change in the quality of health care, health care professionals must utilize leadership principles. Changing behavior is difficult, and there are always multiple barriers to change efforts. To be effective in leading transformation, change efforts need to create a sense of urgency, be data-driven, team-based, specific, and measurable.

Successful leadership can be achieved even without a formal position of authority. Strategies for effectively influencing change include the following:

- Gathering compelling data
- Adopting a 'systems' view of the problem
- Getting buy-in from administrative leadership or a powerful clinicalally
- Developing ideas to solve the problem
- Formulating an action plan

Goals should be SMART (**s**pecific, **m**easurable, **a**chievable, **r**ealistic, and **t**ime-sensitive). Good leaders are able to organize a team, articulate clear goals, manage conflict resolution, and make decisions based on the input of team members. Good leaders also lead by example and model good patient safety behavior.

KEY DEFINITIONS

- **Adverse event:** any injury caused by medical care
  - An adverse event results in unintended harm to a patient by an act of commission or omission, rather than by the underlying disease or condition of the patient. Identifying something as an adverse event does not imply error, negligence, or poor quality care. It simply indicates that an undesirable clinical outcome resulted from some aspect of diagnosis or therapy, not an underlying disease process.
- **Adverse reaction:** occurs when unexpected harm results from a justified action
  - An adverse drug reaction occurs when the correct process was followed for the context in which the medication was used.
- **Authority gradient**: command hierarchy of power or balance of power, measured in terms of steepness
  - First used in aviation to describe the phenomenon where pilots and copilots failed to communicate effectively in stressful situations due to the significant difference in their perceived expertise or authority.

Hierarchies which exist in medicine are also subject to causing errors. Most health care teams require some degree of authority gradient; otherwise roles are blurred and decisions cannot be made in a timely fashion. However, within a hierarchy, tools of effective clinical communication and teamwork can overcome risks to patient safety.

- **Brief**: short planning session prior to the start of a clinical activity, in order to achieve team orientation, establish expectations, anticipate problems, and plan for contingencies
- **Checklist**: algorithmic listing of actions to be performed in a given clinical setting, with the goal to ensure that no critical step will be forgotten
  - Though a seemingly simple intervention, checklists have played a leading role in the most significant successes of the patient safety movement, including the near-elimination of central line–associated bloodstream infections in many intensive care units. Checklists have also been used in the operating room to ensure that OR teams are well-oriented and that evidence-based standards known to reduce complications are followed (e.g. use of pre-operative antibiotics).
- **Closed-loop communication:** a type of communication whereby, when a request is made of team members, someone specifically affirms out loud that he or she will complete the task and states out loud when the task has been completed
  - For example, during a cardiac resuscitation a physician orders a medication to be given intravenously and the nurse verbally confirms receipt of the order and verbally confirms when the medication has been administered as requested.
- **Debrief:** information exchange process designed to improve team performance and effectiveness, held after a clinical event in order to review and learn
- **Error**: failure of a planned action to be completed as intended or the use of a wrong plan to achieve an aim (i.e. an act of commission or doing something wrong); also includes failure of an unplanned action that should have been completed (i.e. an act of omission, or failing to do the right thing)
  - For example, ordering a medication for a patient with a documented allergy to that medication is an error of commission. Failing to prescribe a proven medication with major benefits for an eligible patient (e.g. low-dose unfractionated heparin for venous thromboembolism prophylaxis for a patient after hip replacement surgery) is an **error of omission**.Errors of omission are more difficult to recognize than errors of commission but are thought to represent a larger scope of the problem in patient safety. Errors can also be defined in terms of active or latent as coined by Professor James Reason, one of the founders in the field of safety science. According to Professor Reason, **active errors** occur at the point of contact between a human and some aspect of a larger system (e.g., a human–machine interface). They are generally readily apparent (e.g., pushing an incorrect button, ignoring a warning light) and almost always involve someone at the frontline. Active errors or active failures are sometimes referred to as

errors at the 'sharp end,' figuratively referring to a scalpel. In other words, errors at the sharp end are noticed first because they are committed by the person closest to the patient. This person may literally be holding a scalpel (e.g., an orthopedist operating on the wrong leg) or figuratively be administering any kind of therapy (e.g., a nurse programming an intravenous pump with the wrong medication dose) or performing any aspect of care.
Latent errors (or latent conditions), in contrast, refer to less apparent failures of organization or design that contribute to the occurrence of errors or allow them to cause harm to patients. To complete the metaphor, latent errors are those at the other end of the scalpel—the 'blunt end'—referring to the many layers of the health care system that affect the person "holding" the scalpel. For example, policies that allow a patient to enter an operating room and start an operation before confirming the patient's identify, intended procedure and site of surgery are considered latent errors that can result in wrong patient or wrong site surgery.

- **Forcing function**: aspect of a design which prevents a specific action from being performed or allows its performance only if another specific action is performed first
  - For example, automobiles are now designed so that the driver cannot shift into reverse without first putting a foot on the brake pedal. One of the first forcing functions identified in health care was the removal of concentrated potassium from general hospital wards. This action is intended to prevent the inadvertent preparation of intravenous solutions with concentrated potassium, an error that had produced small but consistent numbers of deaths for many years.
- **Handoffs**: the process whereby one health care professional updates another on the status of ≥1 patients for the purpose of taking over their care
  - An example includes a resident physician who has been on call overnight telling an incoming resident about the patients admitted who require ongoing management. Nurses commonly conduct a handover at the end of their shift, updating the oncoming nurse about their status of the patients and tasks that need to be performed. Handoffs are a potential source of patient safety failure from the lack of important information being conveyed or misinformation being conveyed.
- **Harm/hazard**: harm is the impairment or any negative effect on the structure of function of the body (e.g., disease, injury, suffering, disability, death); hazard is a circumstance, agent or action with the potential to cause harm
- **Huddle:** an often impromptu problem-solving meeting conducted in order to assess a critical situation, reestablish situation awareness, reinforce plans already in place, and determine the need to adjust the plan
- **Iatrogenic:** an adverse effect of medical care, rather than of the underlying disease (literally "brought forth by healer," from Greek *iatros*, for healer, and *gennan*, to bring forth)

- **Incident reporting**: collecting and analyzing information about an event which could have harmed (near-miss) or did harm (adverse event) a patient in a health care setting
- **Medication error**: any preventable event which may cause or lead to unintended and incorrect medication use or patient harm, while the medication is in the control of the health care professional or patient
  - Medication error occurs when a patient receives (a) the wrong medication, or (b) the right medication but in the wrong dosage or manner (e.g. given orally instead of IV, correct medication given at the wrong time).
- **Medication reconciliation**: process of avoiding unintended inconsistencies in medication regimens which can occur with any transition in care (e.g. hospital admission, transfer to ICU, discharge to rehab center) by reviewing the patient's current medication regimen and comparing it with the regimen being considered for the new setting of care
  - Medical reconciliation helps to ensure that the intended medications are continued, and that medications that are supposed to be discontinued are not inadvertently continued. For example, medical reconciliation performed prior to discharging a patient from the hospital can detect if medication changes were made during the hospital stay that need to be continued once the patent is home (e.g. intravenous antibiotics started in the hospital during the treatment of pneumonia which are intended to be continued orally at home).
- **Near-miss (or close call)**: error or other incident which does not produce patient injury, but only because of intervening factors or pure chance
  - This good fortune might reflect robustness of the patient (e.g., a patient with penicillin allergy receives penicillin, but has no reaction) or a fortuitous, timely intervention (e.g., a nurse happens to realize that a physician wrote an order in the wrong chart).
- **Patient safety**: The WHO defines patient safety as 'the reduction of risk of unnecessary harm associated with health care to an acceptable minimum (2009)
  - The Agency for Healthcare Research and Quality uses the definition that 'patient safety is a discipline in the health care sector that applies safety science methods toward the goal of achieving a trustworthy system of health care delivery. Patient safety is also an attribute of health care systems; it minimizes the incidence and impact of, and maximizes recovery from, adverse events.
- **Quality assurance (QA):** an older term, not likely to be used today; QA was reactive, retrospective, policing, and in many ways punitive; often involved determining who was at fault after something went wrong
- **Quality improvement (QI):** involves both prospective and retrospective reviews; is aimed at improvement— measuring where you are and figuring out ways to make things better; specifically attempts to avoid attributing blame and to create systems to prevent errors from happening
- **Read backs (or call-backs)**: when a listener repeats key information so that the transmitter can confirm its correctness

- To address the possibility of miscommunication when information is conveyed verbally, many high-risk industries use protocols for mandatory read-backs. For example, a laboratory technician calling a physician with a critical lab value may request that the physician read back the critical lab value to ensure it was received correctly.

- **Root cause analysis (RCA):** structured process for identifying the causal or contributing factors underlying adverse events or other critical incidents
  - Initially developed to analyze industrial accidents, RCA is now widely employed in error analysis within health care. A central tenet of RCA is to identify underlying problems that increase the likelihood of errors, while avoiding the trap of focusing on mistakes by individuals. RCA seeks to explore all the possible factors associated with an incident by asking what happened, why it happened, and what can be done to prevent it from happening again.
- **SBAR:** a form of structured communication first developed for use in naval military procedures; it stands for situation (what is going on with the patient?), background (what is the clinical background or context?), assessment (what do I think the problem is?), recommendation/request (what would I do to correct it?)
  - It has been adapted for health care as a helpful technique for communicating critical information that requires immediate attention and action concerning a patient's condition. It promotes patient safety by helping individuals communicate with shared expectations in a concise and structured format which improves efficiency and accuracy.
- **Sentinel event:** adverse event in which death or serious harm to a patient has occurred; used to refer primarily to events that were not at all expected or acceptable (e.g., an operation on the wrong patient or body part)
- **Violation:** intentional or deliberate deviation from safe operating procedures, standards, or policies
  - A violation is different from an error, which is an unintentional action. Unlike errors which are honest mistakes due to human nature, intentional violations are behaviors for which individuals need to be held accountable.
- **Wrong-site procedure**: operation or procedure done on the wrong part of the body or on the wrong person; it can also mean the wrong surgery or procedure was performed
  - Wrong-site procedures are rare and preventable, though they do still occur. A standard system to confirm the patient, site, and intended procedure with the medical team and patient before starting the procedure is a widely employed method of reducing or eliminating wrong-site procedures.

Review Questions

1. A 64-year-old man is admitted to the hospital for treatment of bacterial pneumonia. The treating clinician forgets to ask about allergies and the patient is unaware that his severe allergy to penicillin is not known to the treatment team. The patient receives a dose of intravenous penicillin and suffers an anaphylactic response but is successfully resuscitated by the medical team. Which of the following is the most accurate description of the medical error?

   A. Slip resulting in a near miss

   B. Violation resulting in a near miss

   C. Lapse resulting in an adverse event

   D. Violation resulting in patient injury

   E. Non-preventable adverse event

A new intern who is not being supervised is asked to see a patient who is being discharged following treatment of a lower extremity deep vein thrombosis. The intern prescribes a six month course of warfarin without reviewing the patient's other medications. Unknown to the intern, the patient is taking an antibiotic which increases the anticoagulant activity of warfarin. The pharmacy computer system is broken and the drug is filled manually, which does not enable the computer system to alert to the drug –drug interaction. An overworked nurse fails to check for drug interactions during the medication reconciliation and gives the patient the prescription upon discharge. The patient fills the prescription at a local drug store and suffers a significant bleeding complication requiring re-hospitalization and surgery.

2. According to James Reason's Swiss cheese model of error, which one of the following would be the most effective approach to preventing this adverse event in the future?

   A. Identifying and correcting the single overarching failure in the health care system responsible for the adverse event

   B. Identifying and weeding out the individuals involved in this medical error

   C. Applying a systemic approach to eliminating all causes of human error

   D. Building successive layers of safety barriers into the system that prevent medical error from resulting in patient harm

   E. Initiating a campaign to remind clinicians to be more vigilant and to follow established safety protocols

3. As a member of the clinical team you are interested in developing a new system to more closely monitor blood glucose levels of diabetic patients admitted to the hospital for vascular wound care. In order to assess the impact of this new system on patient quality, you and your team conduct a PDSA cycle. Which of the following statements is correct regarding the PDSA cycle?

   A. The PDSA cycle begins with full scale implementation
   B. The PDSA cycle consists of small, rapid test of new initiatives
   C. Changes from PDSA are based on expert intuition, and do not require data collection or interpretation
   D. PDSA is a means of analyzing past errors in order to design system based interventions
   E. The PDSA cycle requires a randomized control trial

4. A 23-year-old man with a history of depression is admitted to the inpatient psychiatry ward after the third attempt at suicide with an intentional drug overdose. The patient has been stabilized medically; however, is under 24-hour monitoring by the nursing staff due to repeated attempts at self-harm. During change of shift, there is a mistake in communication and no one is assigned to the patient. The mistake is noticed 15 minutes into the new shift, and a member of the nursing team is assigned to watch the patient. Fortunately, during the 15-minute period the patient did not make any attempts to harm himself. Which of the following statements about this event is correct?

   A. This is a sentinel event and should be reported to the medical board
   B. This is a sentinel event and should be reported to the hospital and family
   C. This is a near miss and should be reported to the hospital
   D. This is a near miss and should be reported to the patient and family
   E. This is a near miss and no reporting is required since the patient was not harmed

5. A nurse practitioner receives a phone call from the mother of one of the pediatric patients in the practice who frequently suffers from ear infections. The mother typically sees the physician and receives antibiotics to treat her child's condition. Given that it is a weekend and the office is closed, the nurse practitioner phones in the antibiotic prescription based on the mother's recollection of the name of the medication used in the past. The prescription is filled at a new pharmacy that does not have the patient's prior medical records on file. The child suffers an allergic reaction after which it is discovered that the wrong antibiotic was ordered. Which of the following statements is correct regarding root cause analysis (RCA)?

   A. RCA involves a retrospective, systems approach to error analysis
   B. RCA is a prospective approach to systems redesign
   C. RCA involves only the individual(s) directly involved in the error
   D. RCA is only performed for errors resulting in patient death
   E. Due to privacy laws the results of RCA are confidential and not shared

A critical and respiratory care unit is attempting to decrease their rate of ventilator-acquired pneumonia. The team develops a new clinical protocol to help reduce hospital acquired pneumonia in ventilated patients. The protocol includes several new activities which have not previously been followed uniformly in the unit. The changes includes head of bed elevation, daily oral care, daily assessment of readiness to extubate and having access to infectious disease specialists for consultation in the treatment of ventilator-associated pneumonia.

6. Which one of the following represents an outcomes measure of quality?
   A. Measure the compliance rate in following guidelines for head of bed elevation over a 3 month period following the new protocol
   B. Determine the number of infectious disease specialists available for consultation during a 3 month period following the new protocol.
   C. Monitor the number of patients who self-extubate prematurely during the daily assessment of readiness to extubate over a 3 months period following implementation of the new protocol
   D. Monitor the number of infections over 3 months following implementation of the new protocol
   E. Determine the wait time for starting antibiotics in patients with suspected ventilator-associated pneumonia.

7. A geriatric team is interested in decreasing the number of patient falls in their nursing home. After convening as a group to discuss possible interventions, a new system of identifying patients at high-risk for falling and providing these patients with fall prevention interventions is implemented. Following this intervention, the rate of patient falls per month is followed for 12 months on a run chart. No baseline data was collected. Which of the following best describes the results of the run chart?

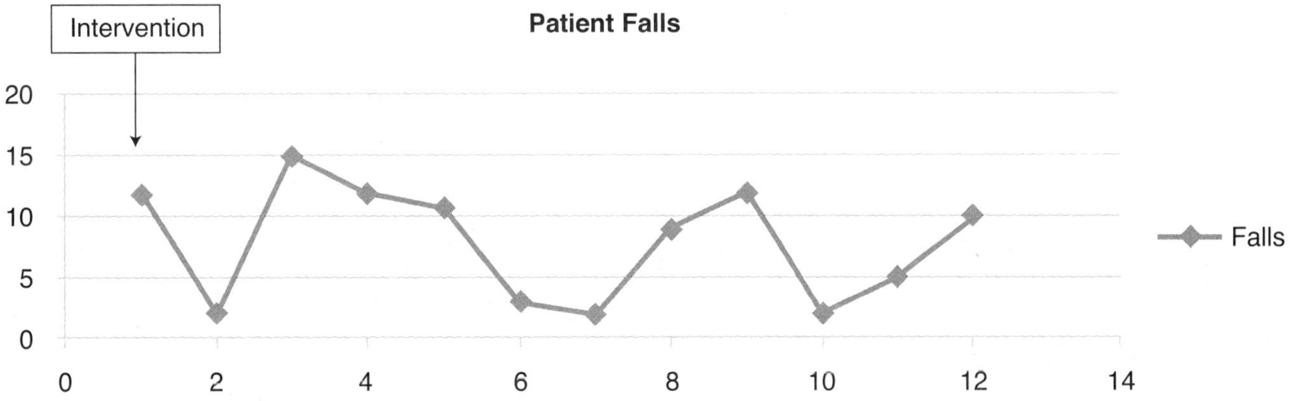

   A. The intervention led to a significant decrease in patient falls
   B. The intervention led to a significant increase in patient falls
   C. The intervention resulted in no change in patient falls
   D. The impact of the intervention is subjective
   E. The impact of the intervention is inconclusive

8. An 85-year-old woman is being transferred to an acute rehabilitation facility following a hospital admission for hip replacement surgery. Postoperatively during her hospital stay she was started on deep vein thrombosis (DVT) prophylaxis medication with plans to continue the medication upon discharge. The intern and nurse discharging the patient failed to convey this new medication to the receiving treatment team at the rehabilitation center. The patient is not continued on her anticoagulation medication and sustains a DVT leading to a fatal pulmonary embolus 3 weeks after transfer. Which of the following actions will facilitate quality improvement and the prevention of a similar error in the future?

   A. Determine which staff member(s) failed to order the medication
   B. Develop a process to increase the use of medication reconciliation
   C. Send a memo to all staff about the importance of DVT prophylaxis
   D. Educate patients about the dangers of DVT following hip surgery
   E. Conduct monthly audits to monitor medication errors at transitions of care

Answers and Explanations

1. **Answer: C.** A lapse is an internal event that generally involves a failure in memory; as opposed to a slip which is an observable action commonly associated with attentional or perceptional failures resulting in an unintended execution of a correctly intended action. The result of the described error was harm to the patient in the form of anaphylaxis with the need for resuscitation, and therefore is categorized as an adverse event. An adverse event is any harm or undesirable clinical outcome resulting from medical care as opposed to the underlying disease process, and does not have to result in permanent disability or death. A violation is a deliberate act of not following policy or procedures, which was not the situation in this scenario. A near miss is an event or a situation that does not produce patient harm, but only because of intervening factors or good fortune. The adverse event described is the result of an error and is completely preventable.

2. **Answer: D.** The most effective approach to improving patient safety and quality is to address system-level causes of failure. In the Swiss-cheese model, safety barriers are recognized as having unintended weaknesses (i.e. holes) which can occasionally align and allow an error to result in patient harm. In order to improve patient safety, the system must be redesigned to have effective safety barriers capable of preventing errors from resulting in patient harm. Attempting to penalize individuals who make honest errors or eliminate the potential for human error yields limited results.

3. **Answer: B.** The PDSA Cycle is a systematic series of steps for gaining valuable learning and knowledge for the continual improvement of a product or process The PDSA cycle consists of developing a plan to test an intervention (Plan), carrying out the intervention (Do), observing and measuring the impact of the intervention (Study), and determining what modifications should be made to the system or process as a result of the study observations (Act). These interventions are small scale, rapid tests of new initiatives. Interventions with promising results are then selected for larger scale implementation. They do not require the rigor of random-

ized controlled trials. These 4 steps are repeated over and over as part of a never-ending cycle of continual improvement.

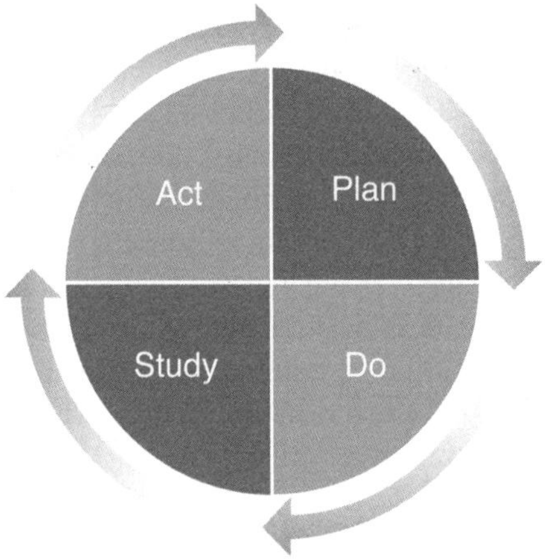

4. **Answer: C.** The event described is a near miss; there was an error which fortunately did not result in patient harm. Most near misses need not be disclosed to patients or families; however, they should be reported to the hospital in order for the error to be studied in an attempt to learn how to prevent it in the future. A sentinel event is an adverse event resulting in serious or permanent injury to a patient.

5. **Answer: A.** The root cause analysis is a retrospective approach to error analysis. It is typically performed for errors resulting in significant patient harm, but can be performed for any adverse event that a team wishes to review. The RCA process usually involves the individual(s) involved in the event as well as any other members of the team typically involved in the care delivery process related to the event. Although the details such as the names of the individuals involved in the event are not shared publically, the general findings of the RCA can be shared throughout the system in order to improve the quality of the system.

6. **Answer: D.** The number of infections over 3 months following implementation of the new protocol is an outcomes measure. Compliance rates in following guidelines are a process measure. The number of infectious disease specialists would be a structure measure. The number of patients prematurely self-extubating would be a balancing measure. Wait times for starting antibiotics is another process measure.

7. **Answer: E.** A run chart provides a dynamic display of a process over time. Run charts help to determine using minimal mathematical complexity if interventions made in a process or system over time lead to improvements. Run charts also provide the foundation for the more sophisticated method of statistical analysis using control charts. The run chart allows a team to understand the stability of a process as well as determine any shifts, trends or runs which may indicate changes based on interventions. However, without a baseline for comparison, one cannot determine from this run chart whether or not any significant change has occurred.

8. **Answer: B.** Quality assurance (QA) is an older term describing a process that is reactive and retrospective in nature. It is a form of 'policing' to ensure that quality standards have been followed. It often relies on audits and traditionally has focused on punitive actions for failures in quality. It often involved determining who was at fault after something went wrong. QA has not proven to be very effective in transforming care. The goal of quality improvement (QI), on the other hand, is to achieve improvement by measuring the current status of care and then developing systems-based approaches to making things better. It involves both prospective and retrospective reviews and specifically attempts to avoid attributing blame. Rather, QI seeks to create systems to prevent errors from happening. In the case above, developing a process to increase the use of medication reconciliation would be following the principles of QI. The other interventions are QA-based and/or simply not as effective in creating and sustaining a positive change.

Index

D

E

I

K

Q

R

S

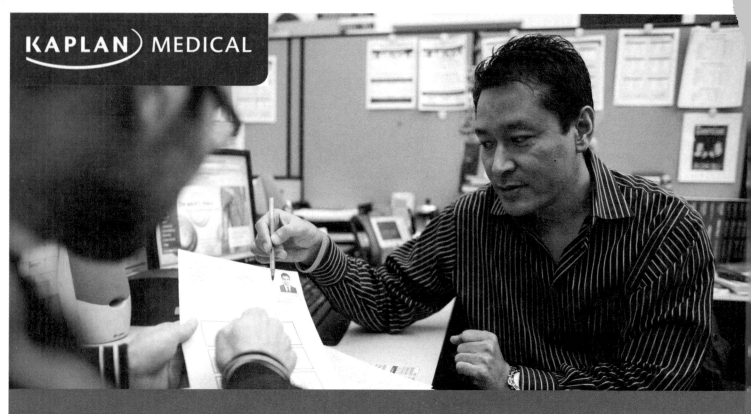